The
YOGURT
DIET

The
YOGURT
DIET

The Real Secret to
Good Health,
Ideal Weight
and Long Life

Ana Luque

Salud Life, LLC

Los Angeles   London   Barcelona

US- 310. 765.4089

EU- 011.34.93.802.1340

myyogurtdiet.com

For information about wholesale purchases, please contact our sales department at any of the numbers above

Text and recipes Copyright © 2008 Ana Luque

Photography by Shawn Frederick

Book Cover and Layout Design by Dan C. Gomez

Manufactured in the United States of America

10   9   8   7   6   5   4   3   2

Library of Congress Cataloging-in-Publication Data has been applied for.

First United States of America printing, September 2008

Luque, Ana

The Yogurt Diet: the real secret to good health, ideal weight and long life

by Ana Luque with Bill Gutman

Includes biographical references. Does not include index.

1. Yogurt.   2. Weight Loss.   3. Health and Fitness.   4. Probiotics.

ISBN 978-0-615-24105-0

For Steve,
My best friend.

You are the light that guides my path so that I never get lost,
the hand that holds mine tight so that I never fall,
the soothing voice that makes my fears disappear,
and the encouraging presence in my life who doesn't allow me
to be anything less than extraordinary.

Your noble heart, unconditional friendship, altruistic kindness
and dedicated mentorship create magic in the lives of all you
touch. You are an inspiration for a better world.

Hope is like a road in the country; there was never a road, but when many people walk on it, the road comes into existence.

— Lin Yutang (Chinese writer)

May The Yogurt Diet be the book that unravels the many answers to end the obesity epidemic and brings hope to those who, despite of debilitating illnesses, embrace life with grace and courage.

Acknowledgments

Writing this book has been a beautiful journey that could have not been traveled without the love, support and knowledge of the following friends.

Bill Gutman, my devoted writing partner and mentor, who believed in me without reservations and took me under his wing to write my first book.

Tim Clegg, CEO of Americhip, a true leader, who is committed to bringing out the best in people. He has taught me the precious lesson that when one relates to the dreams of others, you empower them to make their dreams possible. This book is proof of that.

Fidel Arizmendi, who introduced me to Mexico and its enchanting culture, something that has radically transformed my life. Also, for his inspiration to reconnect to my Spanish roots and teaching me to give my heart fully to everything I do in life.

Mom and Dad, who devoted their lives to creating infinite magic, love and beauty for their children and who have, without judgment, always been an empowering force for us to follow our dreams.

More Acknowledgments

Dr. Palani, DDS, who contributed his knowledge to the writing of this book. For his continued dedication to deliver painless and holistic dental care to his patients, and for raising awareness of the great importance of yogurt for oral health. His diligent devotion to his patients illuminates the world with healthy and beautiful smiles everyday.

Russell, for your wonderful notes on the very first draft of this book, which set me on the right path and have made this book that much better. You and **Daryl** have a very special place in my heart. **David Botfeld,** may the Yogurt Diet bring out all the sexiness in you! Thank you for everything. **Jessica Junyent,** I can't thank you enough for your great contributions throughout the writing of this book. You are the best girlfriend a girl could ask for. **Dr. Ravins,** for your continued support and belief in me.

I would like to especially acknowledge all the scientists and doctors who give their lives to the research of probiotics, because without them this book would have not been possible. And my special thanks to **Natasha Trenev** of Natren Probiotics, for her tireless dedication to raise awareness to the public of the importance of probiotics for human health. Her books are a precious contribution to the world.

If more friends like these existed, everyone's life would be filled with magic and the possibility of greatness would be attainable in each and all of us.

Contents

Chapter Four

Chapter Five

Chapter Six

Chapter Seven

My Love Affair with Yogurt

I grew up in Spain where, as in so many other parts of the world, milk-fermented foods are a staple of the national diet and are consumed daily in the form of yogurt, kefir, butter and cheese. Some of my happiest memories stem from my childhood, with so many of them revolving around delicious foods and being surrounded by loving family and friends. One of my most cherished moments from those days was coming home from school and sitting outside on the porch with mom, my sister and two brothers. We would share our adventures of the day while each eating a bowl of natural, homemade creamy yogurt with a thick layer of raw honey dripping on top. That was magnificent in itself! But the final touch of adding crumbs of Maria cookies to this mountain of "yumminess" made it a snack that was out of this world – the perfect combination of creaminess, sweetness and crispiness. Is there any dessert more delicious than that? To us as kids it was like eating the most decadent of junk foods! But mom knew she had us fooled in the right way because we were really eating the most perfect food possible. Yogurt.

To this day yogurt remains my biggest treat. I will choose yogurt with honey, seasonal fruits and nuts over any other dessert in the world. In fact, not a single day passes by that I don't eat yogurt at least once. It not only continues to taste wonderful, but I am now fully aware of the many healthful benefits it brings to my body. It keeps me fit, healthy, youthful and always unstoppable.

At one time yogurt was considered a luxury food, one not available to everyone because only a few really knew how to make it. Today, good quality yogurt is widely available at grocery stores and anyone can make it. In the following pages you will hopefully realize that the act of eating yogurt may well be the healthiest dietary decision you can ever make.

-- Ana Luque

Introduction

The Yogurt Diet is far from another of those fad diets that appear on the scene like a comet and flame out just as quickly. This rather simple diet, featuring one of the oldest foods known to man, will provide a means for changing your life and give you the real secret to discovering the magical combination of perfect weight and radiant health. That's right! If you embrace the Yogurt Diet you will absolutely lose weight and never regain it, and you'll enjoy an enriched and healthy life for many, many years to come. Could you ask for better news than that?

In fact, after you've undoubtedly been bombarded with every type of special diet over the years, as well as promises that only seem to bring failure and disappointment, you'll be both surprised and delighted to learn that a real and lasting solution can be so simple. The Yogurt Diet not only reveals the causes of the widespread obesity and disease epidemics that continue to plague our population, but it offers a permanent solution, as well. This is far from a frivolous statement. Believe it or not, yogurt is one of the most heavily researched foods in the world. Because of the well-known variety of beneficial properties contained in yogurt, scientists have now equated its use with a way to counter many common ailments in addition to contributing to the long and healthy life of those who make it a regular staple of their diet.

Yogurt is far from being the new food on the block. It has an extensive history dating back thousands of years, and millions of people from countries all around the globe have consumed this wonder food. Even more startling is new scientific evidence which reveals that the bacteria found in yogurt may very well be the missing link to permanent weight loss. The Yogurt Diet will also reveal how eating yogurt can be the key to developing an all-important, ultra-fast metabolism.

The Yogurt Diet that will be described in this book is designed to be followed safely by any adult, as well as children over the age of two. Its goal will be to allow followers to achieve radiant health, find an ideal weight, and live a long, disease-free life.

As has been the case with so many people who have eaten yogurt over the years, may all of us live to celebrate that magical 100th birthday!

Chapter One

What is Yogurt and Where Did it Come From

In simplest terms, yogurt is the fermentation of milk sugars by specific microbes, namely lactic acid bacteria (LAB). These bacteria break down the sugar lactose into lactic acid (thus, the name lactic acid bacteria), creating an acidic atmosphere in which harmful organisms cannot live. During this process, both the protein and fats in the milk are also partially pre-digested by the bacteria, making the resulting yogurt more digestible and easier for the body to assimilate.

The beneficial bacteria used in yogurt making are Lactobacillus bulgaricus and Streptococcus thermophilus, though other species such as L. acidophilus, Lactobacillus Casei, L. rhamnosus, L. Burgaricus, L. Salivarious; as well as the Bifidobacteria, Bifidobacterium infantis and B. longum are also sometimes added for additional health benefits. All of these bacteria are naturally found in large numbers in the intestines of healthy humans. While the names might seem long and difficult to pronounce, the many health properties they offer are immeasurable. Because these organisms are loaded with a host of life-promoting properties they are often referred to as probiotic bacteria, meaning "for life."

Yogurt is made from the milk of various mammals, thus it has all the properties from an already nutrient-rich natural food. But when the milk is fermented into yogurt it becomes a food far superior to its original form. It is the live active cultures of bacteria that enhance and add the extra health benefits that go well beyond those of fresh milk. For these reasons, probiotic yogurt is considered a perfect food, one that has been associated with long life in every place where it is consumed regularly. In fact, there are still many parts of the world where milk is only consumed in the form of yogurt. Just that fact alone should tell you something, the secret of why these centenarians live such healthy lives

What Are Probiotics?

Probiotics are live microorganisms which, when administered in adequate amounts, confer a health benefit on the host. There's also a population of probiotic bacteria, or "friendly bacteria," naturally living throughout the digestive tract of humans and other animals, which are necessary for life.

Breaking it down to the basics, yogurt is a very good source of calcium, phosphorus, riboflavin/vitamin B-2 and iodine. It is also a good source of protein, vitamin B-12, tryptophan, potassium, pantothenic acid/vitamin B-5, zinc and molybdenum (a necessary mineral). Just having these 11 nutrients alone make yogurt a super food. But when you add the presence of the probiotic bacteria and the healthful wonders they can achieve, then you have a super food that is, in every sense of the word, a true life-promoting product.

Probiotic Bacteria in Yogurt and your Health

Let me say up front that all the health benefits, cures and preventative measures discussed in his book – and attributed to eating yogurt – have scientific backing from doctors and researchers who have been conducting controlled studies for many years and have published their conclusive findings in both medical and nutritional journals. Thus the information contained in this book is considerably more than just one person's opinion.

Now let's get right to it. As shocking as it may sound, rather than just genes, excess calories, unhealthy fats and processed carbohydrates being the sole contributing factors in the cause of obesity and disease, emerging evidence strongly suggest that one more potential factor that will determine your health and body weight is the lack of a healthy gut flora in your digestive tract. In essence, there is an army of friendly bacteria at the forefront of the body's immune system ready to do battle against the invading forces of illness and nutrient-robbing bad bacteria. Not surprisingly, this army of good bacteria – part of the immune system – is made up of many of the same species naturally present in yogurt. It's obvious, then, that we need these kinds of microbes – the probiotics – to live healthy lives. They are an essential component of the body's defense mechanism that protect us against inflammation, which we now know is a major factor in the onset of disease.

Here's what happens. When the friendly bacterial flora in your body becomes depleted or is destroyed – for reasons you will learn later in the book – the immune system becomes compromised and the body begins to experience many symptoms which can lead to possibly dangerous consequences. Among the outcomes hastened by a weak immune system are rapid weight gain and the onset of inflammation, including the following conditions – obesity, chronic fatigue, diabetes, periodontal disease, diarrhea, constipation, Irritable Bowel Syndrome

(IBS), cardiovascular disease, skin disorders , bad breath, attention deficit disorder (ADD), milk intolerance, celiac disease, osteoporosis, infertility, impotence, asthma, slow metabolism, migraines, poor digestion, acid reflux, yeast infections, urinary tract infections, fungus on the nails, ear and nasal infections, chest congestion, arthritis, ulcers, allergies, high blood pressure, cancer and many more.

Microbes Are Everywhere

Microbes or micro-organisms are microscopic, single-celled living organisms, which include bacteria and fungi (yeasts), but not viruses. Microbes live almost everywhere on earth where there is water and, contrary to popular belief, most of them are not harmful.

If you are surprised and taken back by this long list of ailments, stop and think for a minute. Do you have any of these problems? Does anyone in your family complain about them? Perhaps a friend? Or even someone at the office? If that's the case, then the time is right for you to not only read on and share this wonderful information with loved ones, but also to begin following the very delicious and healthful Yogurt Diet.

A Brief History of Yogurt

Yogurt didn't just appear on the scene overnight. In fact, I think it might surprise you to know that the first incidences of yogurt consumption may have indeed happened by accident. The people of the Neolithic Era, living in the Near East around 6000 BC, were among the earliest groups to practice farming and milking their animals. There's a very good chance that they were eating an early form of yogurt. Nomadic herdsmen carried milk in sheepskin bags made from the animals' stomachs, which naturally contain lactic acid bacteria and the enzyme rennin. That environment in combination with the local warm weather would cause the milk to ferment and curdle. And just like that, the earliest form of yogurt was created.

Remember, in those days there was no refrigeration and milk was not pasteurized (a process of sterilization), so fermentation became the best method to preserve milk for long periods of time. Raw milk from mammals (including that of humans) has a natural abundance of probiotic bacterial species, therefore under the right conditions it can be fermented by the naturally occurring beneficial organisms turning the milk into yogurt. It is the acidic environment of yogurt, which prevents spoilage organisms from growing. This simple process makes the fermentation of milk a natural method of pasteurization. But in these early civilizations the fermentation process created yet something else – a food that quickly took on a life of its own. The people from various ancient cultures praised yogurt as a "food from the Gods." It was said that this miraculous substance was made by divine Goddesses to honor their Gods, and that they would feed it daily to them for virility, strength, magnificence and wisdom. At the same time, the Goddesses also consumed yogurt for beauty, purity, fertility and eternal youth. Can you imagine that kind of endorsement on a television commercial today? Yogurt was also popular during the Roman Empire, as well as in ancient Greece and Egypt for its well-documented healthful attributes.

Yogurt, as well as other fermented milk products, has long been a staple in the diets of various cultures of the Middle East, Asia, India, Russia, Eastern Europe and the Mediterranean. It's apparent that yogurt has played an important role in many different world cuisines and, not surprisingly, each has its own name for this universally important and healthful food. In Russia it's called *varenetz*; in Egypt *leben raib*; to the Armenians it's *matzoon*; and in Yugoslavia, where many centenarians live, this creamy delight is known as *kisselo mleko* and sold on street stands as a yummy treat. To the French and Spanish the name will sound a lot more familiar. They simply call it yogurt.

In the early 1900s, yogurt finally began gaining international acclaim thanks to the Russian bacteriologist, Dr. Ilya Ilitch Metchnikov, a pioneer immune system researcher who won the Nobel Prize in 1908. Dr. Metchnikov studied the diets of Bulgarians who lived unusually long lives and soon began speculating that this phenomenon was due to the high consumption of fermented milk products and the ingestion of lactic acid producing bacteria present in these foods. He was also the first to develop a theory that pointed to harmful bacteria in the gut as a cause of aging, and believed strongly that a healthy balance of life promoting gut flora was the key to a long and disease-free life.

In the 1920s, Dr. Minouri Shirota, concerned about the high death rate among children in his native Japan due to infectious diseases and malnutrition, set on a quest to find ways to prevent this problem. During his research, he learned about the various people in the Mediterranean, Eastern Europe and other parts of the world who, by consuming yogurt daily, had a low incident of disease and lived long lives. He then discovered a type of healthful bacteria – namely lactic acid bacteria – in human intestines which not only destroy harmful organisms, but were also responsible for preventing many diseases and could promote a long and healthy life. It was his research that eventually led to the increased consumption of yogurt in Japan, even though milk was not a staple of their traditional diet.

And it was a health conscious and ambitious entrepreneur from Barcelona, fully aware of the health benefits of fermented milk, who first commercialized yogurt in 1919 and made it a staple in the diets of the Spanish people. Today, Spaniards enjoy yogurt as dessert after meals or as a delicious snack with lots of raw honey and nuts, making them one of the largest consumers of yogurt in the world. As a native of Spain, it's no wonder to me that my grandparents are more than 100 years old!

Kefir, Another Great Probiotic

Although this is a book about the amazing health properties of yogurt, it would be remiss of me to write an entire book about this wonder food and not introduce its close cousin, kefir, which is another miraculous probiotic that offers very similar health benefits. Kefir is a fermented milk drink, which is believed to have originated in the Caucasus region, the mountains that separate Asia from Europe. Many people there also live well past 100. Researchers attribute the longevity of these people and their ability to reproduce until late in life to the consumption of fermented milk foods with probiotic bacteria.

Traditionally, kefir is prepared by fermenting cow, goat or sheep's milk at room temperature overnight. The kefir grains are a complex combination of beneficial yeasts and bacteria in a clustered environment of proteins, sugars and fats, giving it the appearance of sticky white rice. This combination of life promoting micro-organisms and nutrients present in kefir offers many of the health benefits that are also associated with yogurt, as they share some of the same bacteria of the Lactobacillus and Streptococcus species. In areas of the world where kefir is consumed daily, the grains are given as a gift to loved ones with wishes for a healthy and long life.

While a good quality yogurt is easy to find on the refrigerated shelves of supermarkets across the country, finding real kefir can be more challenging because it has never attained the popularity of its probiotic cousin. However, you should be able to find good quality kefir on the refrigerator section of many health food stores. Kefir's effervescent and lightly acidic taste is wonderful, and the health benefits are invaluable. It is well worth going out of your way to seek this marvelous drink. Then you can alternate kefir with yogurt, getting the best of both worlds with these two miraculous foods.

An Easy Yogurt Recipe

Homemade yogurt is effortless to make, while the flavor and texture are absolutely sublime. To make yogurt you will need very few gadgets, and I'm almost sure that all of the necessary utensils may already be in your kitchen – a double boiler, a long wooden spoon and an oven with a light. Believe it or not, that's it! The reason why you need a double boiler is to bring the milk to a boil. You should not boil the milk in a pot directly in contact with dry heat, as the high temperature will burn the milk and it will scorch in the bottom. This is not something you want.

Even to this day, with as much yogurt as I make for myself, as well as for friends and family, I still improvise my own double boiler. This is how I do it. I fill up a large pot half way with water, and then I place one large glass bowl inside the pot, making sure that the water doesn't go over when it starts boiling; then I add the milk.

Are You Ready?

Now that you have a brief understanding of yogurt and its history, it's time to become familiar with the probiotic bacteria that live in your digestive tract and which are also found in yogurt. These healthy bacteria have been the subject of much debate and curiosity in the health field for a long time, and now have been scientifically proven as essential for life.

1-quart (1 liter) whole milk (non-homogenized preferred)
3 tablespoons live active culture yogurt or one 5 ounce starter
    package freeze dried bacteria

Directions
Improvise a double boiler. Fill up the bowl with whole milk and bring just to a boil. Stir frequently to prevent a layer from forming on the top.
Set aside and let cool off to about 110°F, stirring occasionally to prevent a film from forming. At this time mix in the starter together with one cup of the lukewarm milk and 3 tablespoons natural live active yogurt and pour back into the rest of the milk. If you're using a freeze-dried culture, follow directions on the package.
Preheat oven at 350°F for just 5 minutes. Turn the oven off, insert the bowl of milk and turn the oven light on. This will be your improvised incubator. Leave undisturbed between 6-8 hours. Do not move or insert anything inside, or the delicate fermentation process will get interrupted. Refrigerate for 5 hours before serving. If you opt for a yogurt maker instead, use as directed.

Chapter Two

Good Bacteria –
Probiotics for Life

Every night after dinner while growing up, we would always eat yogurt with delicious fresh fruits for desert. Not a single night passed by back then without mom giving the kids a small bowl of homemade creamy yogurt. She would add seasonal fruits and mix them into the white fluffy clouds of cool yogurt. Then came our favorite part. We would let a spoonful of honey drip over the yogurt, making swirls, and this delicious creation was then completed with a touch of crushed pistachios or pine nuts sprinkled on top. It not only looked beautiful, but eating it was like heaven to me. Some nights my brother, Ivan, would be difficult and refuse to eat the yogurt dessert. So Mom, instead of forcing the yogurt onto Ivan, would tell us a story.

"Dad has a good friend by the name of Pepe, and he is as strong as Superman," she'd say. "Pepe works for a yogurt company and eats lots of yogurt every day. He loves it. And do you know that Pepe became so strong from eating yogurt that he can lift a car off the ground with just his own two hands. That's how strong he is."

No matter how many times we heard the story about this legendary man, the mystic Pepe, we were always in awe of his super powers. "With his own bare hands?" we would ask, admiringly.

And Mom would always respond, "Yes, with his own bare hands. He has arms as big as tanks."

As if this was too good to be true, in unison we would then reply, "Just from eating yogurt?"

"Yes, just from eating yogurt," Mom would confirm. "Pepe is also very old."

Then we would ask, "Older than grandpa?"

"Yes, much, much older than grandpa. But grandpa eats lots of yogurt also, so he too will live to be very old."

By the time she had finished wowing us with her story we had all licked clean our bowl of yogurt and were ready to go play before going to bed.

I may not be able to lift up a car with my own bare hands, but her story was symbolic for the miracle properties I now know yogurt to have. Yes, its properties are truly miraculous. Yogurt, with its probiotic bacteria, can prevent disease and boost the immune system and, as scientists are beginning to discover, even cure illnesses once though incurable. Yogurt is also the secret why the people of the Mediterranean, as well as other parts of the world, stay slim throughout their lives.

The Importance of Friendly Bacteria in the Gut

When you eat yogurt the lactic acid bacteria travel through the digestive tract, establishing colonies on the mucus walls of your intestines and also passing through, as transient, performing and aiding in digestion as well as contributing to other healthful bodily functions. As mentioned earlier, the word probiotic derives from the Greek word pro and biotic. Together they mean for life. We need them because they're essential – no surprise here – for life. You have a symbiotic relationship with the colonies of probiotic bacteria that make your body their home because you need each other to live healthy long lives. The better care you take of them; the better they will take care of you.

Digestive Tract
(Gastrointestinal Tract)

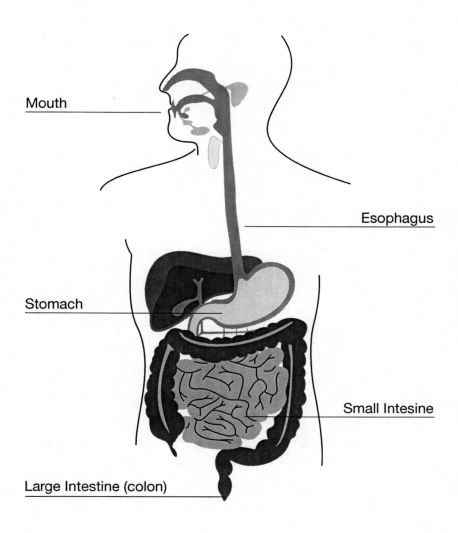

Mouth

Esophagus

Stomach

Small Intesine

Large Intestine (colon)

The fermentation of foods by the lactic acid bacteria (LAB) that live in your gut is a means for these types of beneficial organisms to obtain food and energy. Just as we do, probiotic bacteria also require amino acids, vitamins, minerals, fatty acids and carbohydrates to thrive. This is something to always keep in mind when you're eating, because it is with wholesome foods that you nourish the good microbes in your digestive tract and keep them working their miracles for a lifetime. A diet full of sugar, corn syrup, highly processed carbohydrates, antibiotic and hormone laden animal proteins, pasteurized fruit juices and too much alcohol – basically most processed foods on the shelves of supermarkets today – combine to starve and kill your healthy gut flora and instead promote the growth of harmful organisms in your gut.

You Won't Overeat

Another fabulous benefit of probiotic bacteria living in your digestive tract is that they have also been assigned the job of regulating caloric intake by signaling to the brain that you have had enough to eat. This prevents excess eating and unnecessary food cravings. Think about what a wonderful benefit that can be.

Essentially, what happens during lactic acid fermentation in the digestive tract is the pre-digestion of foods by probiotic bacteria, which in turn produce digestive enzymes that make foods easier for us to digest while also enhancing their nutritional value. This process allows for some vitamins and minerals to become more readily available to the human body, and clearly shows why your friendly little guys play a major role in your health.

The gut micro-flora is responsible for building a fully developed and competent immune system. Bacteria grow in colonies around the mucous membranes of your gastrointestinal tract, acting as a first line of defense to prevent illness by keeping damaging elements from spreading to the rest of your body. The lactic acid produced by LAB possess anti-microbial activities which defend your body from harmful living organisms that enter daily in foods you eat, the water you drink and the air you breath. This is the exact same mechanism used when probiotic bacteria ferment sugars, proteins and fats present in milk, producing an acidic environment that prevents spoilage organisms from growing, thus giving yogurt its long shelf life naturally, without the addition of chemicals and man-made preservatives.

Consuming yogurt regularly is a primary way to restore the much-needed colonies of healthy bacteria in your digestive tract, especially since they are depleted daily. The intestinal flora not only aid in digestion, but also act as a defensive barrier between the outside world and your entire body. Among other benefits, they are responsible for stopping allergens, microbes and other toxins from damaging the mucus membranes that line many areas on the inside of your body, while also preventing harmful substances that can cause illness from entering the blood stream. Adding probiotic yogurt to the diet has proven to be highly effective in reducing or eliminating the effects of certain allergies, such as eczema, lactose intolerance, celiac disease, asthma, and others, while probiotic bacteria can also alleviate symptoms of inflammatory bowel disease. The intestinal flora is responsible for producing important substances, some of which cannot be acquired through diet, but are essential for optimum health. At this point it should be crystal clear how important it is to maintain a good balance of probiotic bacteria in your body to promote excellent health and ideal weight.

How These Guys Set Up Shop in Your Body

In the womb, a baby's intestines are believed to be sterile, meaning there are no live organisms present. The gut flora begins to colonize the digestive system and other parts of the body during the first few weeks of a baby's life and, by age two, the entire ecosystem is well established in the body. When a baby is born naturally through the mother's birth canal, he has the first chance to begin populating his digestive system with some probiotic bacteria that the healthy mother harbors in the vagina. For this reason, it is extremely important that the mother has a balanced bacterial fauna when the baby is born. On the other hand, if the mother has a bacterial or yeast infection in the vagina at the time her baby is born, these will be the first organisms to colonize the baby's digestive tract, resulting in a colicky baby with a possibly compromised immune system, which can lead to a list of health problems. Unfortunately, this imbalance can have lifelong effects if not soon addressed.

Another way a newborn baby acquires a good dose of healthy bacteria is through the mother's breast milk because it's so rich in probiotic bacteria, specifically Bifidobacteria. While a healthy breast fed baby's intestinal flora is 90 percent Bifidobacteria, studies show that this is not the case with bottle-fed babies, who run a high risk for diarrhea as well as for developing allergies and other illnesses. Needless to say, breastfeeding is absolutely necessary for babies to build a strong immune system from the beginning.

It has been proven that babies who begin their lives breast feeding have stronger immune systems and are sick less often than bottle fed babies. They also do not develop allergies as commonly as babies who are fed formula. Finally, a baby establishes the initial probiotic gut flora through the environmental organisms present. Depending on diet and what bacteria exist in the area, babies will have a distinct variety of microbes colonizing their bodies.

For all these reasons it is extremely important for a baby to establish colonies of probiotic bacteria in its digestive tract to develop a strong immune system immediately. Contrary to popular belief, a baby should not be kept sterile, be constantly cleaned and its body disinfected with antibacterial products. If you do this it can prevent the baby's body from building a strong immune system because it will not be exposed to the wide variety of bacteria that naturally coexist in the environment, good or bad, during the most important years of the baby's life. This "hygiene hypothesis" was presented in a conference at the Harvard Medical School, called "Probiotics and the Hygiene Hypothesis: A case for Protective Nutrients." It puts into perspective the rise of immune disorders in developed countries at the same time infectious diseases have declined. There is mounting evidence that the increase in immune disorders is caused by the decreased microbial exposure due to vaccinations, improved hygiene and antibiotics. All of these factors can lead to abnormal responses to allergens. Consequently, the report recommends consuming probiotic bacteria, present in yogurt, to reinforce the immune response of the immune system and reverse the autoimmune disease trend we face in developed countries today.

Gut Flora –
The Missing Piece in the Obesity Puzzle

In recent years, one of the most exciting findings regarding the probiotic gut flora has been the major role they play in obesity, and the conclusion that they may constitute the final missing piece in the disconcerting obesity puzzle. You're probably already asking yourself, "Hey, how can the presence or lack of presence of certain types of microbes influence my weight?" This intriguing and definitive question will be answered throughout the pages of this book. The Yogurt Diet will explain in great detail why this is so, and will open your eyes to a world of well-being that you didn't know existed.

Although there are hundreds of varieties of bacteria living in the human gut, as well as in the gastrointestinal (GI) tract of other mammals, these microbes can all be classified within two major groups – Bacteroides and Firmicutes. Scientists have recently discovered that the microbes in the Bacteroides family are far less abundant in the intestines of obese individuals than in the intestines of their thin counterparts. And by contrast, Firmicutes organisms are present in large numbers in obese people, but in much smaller amounts in thin people.

This clearly gives you a simple overview of what you are about to learn, and how the Yogurt Diet can answer the dietary questions you've always been asking yourself. The lack of probiotic bacteria in the GI tract may very well be the most significant absence in our modern lives, not only as the missing link to the obesity puzzle, but also as part of the sweeping epidemic that is leading to the long list of diseases we are acquiring today. The Yogurt Diet may very well be the miracle solution that you've been searching for over the years.

And to once again point out the importance and necessity of having the right gut flora in your body, many scientists are now referring to it as the microbiota organ. Yes, just like the heart, liver or kidneys, this component of your body performs so many important functions that it is just as essential as the other organs in your body. Only now are we beginning to scratch the surface, learning the health benefits that these species of intestinal microflora provide to us. The biggest stars in the probiotic world are the bacterial species Lactobacillus, Bifidoacterium and Streptococcus. These are the names getting all the recognition these days, and the ones making the headlines in the probiotic world. Not surprisingly, these are the probiotic bacteria that abound in both yogurt and kefir.

How to Buy Probiotic Yogurt

Now that you know some of the miraculous health and weight loss promoting benefits of probiotic bacteria present in yogurt, you might be wondering if all yogurts are created equal and which one is the best. A good quality yogurt should be made from whole milk derived from naturally raised animals whenever possible. The list of ingredients should include nothing more than milk and probiotic bacteria, also known as live active cultures. Other milk-derived products, such as cream, are acceptable. If sugar, corn syrup, preservatives and colorants appear on the list of ingredients, it means that the yogurt you're buying is of lesser quality and probably doesn't contain the same health benefits. A good rule of thumb is the shorter the ingredient list, the better it is for you. Yogurt with fruits likely indicates that sugar has also been added as a preservative. If you desire fruit flavor and sweetness, mix in fresh seasonal fruits and add a touch of the natural sweetener agave. The label should also confirm that the yogurt contains live active cultures and, with some products, the names of the probiotic bacteria will be listed. A yogurt made with whole milk is always best. This bit of controversy will be explained later, so hold on to the thought.

Understanding the Yogurt Diet

My utmost desire when I started researching the Yogurt Diet was to find a solution to end the obesity and disease epidemics that have proliferated in our modern times due mainly to poor nutrition and lack of a healthy relationship with food. The Yogurt Diet has been carefully formulated with many people in mind – those who suffer from ailments such as obesity, localized stubborn weight, diabetes, high cholesterol, skin disorders, celiac disease, lactose intolerance, eating disorders, gum disease, hormone imbalances, ADD, heartburn, migraines, infertility, impotence, autoimmune disorders, IBS, ulcers and colitis, etc. The goal when you embrace the Yogurt Diet is to achieve overall balance that will lead to ideal weight and radiant health. It is, in fact, as much a preventative measure as it can be a cure to many disorders. I hope to teach everyone how to live a healthier, more balanced and fulfilling life through wholesome delicious foods and the well-researched miracle effects of probiotic yogurt. The Yogurt Diet is about achieving balance within every system of the body, so that it can reorganize itself and begin working optimally, with natural weight loss being part of the wonderful side effects.

The following chapters will carefully explain why certain foods promote uncontrollable cravings and eventually lead to disease. You will learn why the body falls out of harmony and how, with the Yogurt Diet, it is possible to bring it back into balance without expensive drugs, diet pills, and chemical laden potions. The Yogurt Diet will open your eyes to the causes of many diseases, and it will teach you that most ailments stem from the same root problem – a weakened immune system due to a lack of healthy bacterial flora in your digestive tract. You will also learn that simply by boosting your immune system and bringing harmony back into the body with a combination of natural foods and three servings of yogurt a day, many ailments are not only preventable but also, in many instances, curable. When a body is unbalanced disease has an open invitation to run rampant, and even certain foods that you may think are healthy may actually be promoting disease in your body.

The immediate goal of the Yogurt Diet is to purify and replenish the body in order to bring it back into harmony. When eating a specific list of wholesome foods and yogurt, and while avoiding other offending foods, the body naturally finds its own balance and that will also lead to effortless weight loss. This simple diet can accomplish that lofty goal in two ways:

1. Before you lose weight, it is of major importance to cleanse internally by eliminating pathogenic substances and organisms that can take over the body's various systems, causing inflammation and weakening the defenses of the immune system.

2. As the body detoxifies it is absolutely imperative to replenish it by reintroducing vitamins and minerals, re-establishing a healthy gut flora through its probiotic properties, and restocking all the enzymes needed for proper digestion and metabolism.

The objective when detoxifying is to purify and repair all organs in the body so that all systems function properly – including the immune, endocrine and metabolic systems – thus allowing it all to work in unison once again. This will not only restore health, but will also allow the body to find its ideal weight naturally.

In a nutshell, the Yogurt Diet will give you the knowledge and tools you need to achieve optimum health and weight. It's a diet with which you'll still be able to eat a delicious array of natural foods so that you'll never feel deprived or hungry, while at the same time adding the magic properties of probiotic yogurt. Eating this miraculous food will help you colonize the walls of your GI tract with a healthy bacterial fauna and replenish enzymes in your digestive system, which undoubtedly have become depleted during years of abuse, including the eating of processed foods, drinking alcohol, taking antibiotics and other drugs, lack of sleep, stress and aging. At the same time, your immune system will be restored so that it works at maximum efficiency to fight disease and obesity.

You Can Do It!

Now that you have been introduced face-to-face to the friendly probiotic bacteria that live inside your GI tract and have a more concise
idea of the astonishing benefits these little guys can offer to help weight
loss and regain health, there are no more excuses why you shouldn't
be radiantly healthy, insanely energetic, and possess the fabulous body
you have always dreamed about. To achieve this simply requires that
you start incorporating yogurt into your diet while following the other
guidelines that are part of the Yogurt Diet. Do that and you'll be well
on your way to achieving your goals. You can do it!

Chapter Three

The Causes of the Obesity Epidemic

For years, experts have offered every solution on the planet for one of the most crucial questions of the twenty-first century. How can the populations of nearly every country achieve good health and ideal weight? The answers offered so far have come at a high cost and have mostly resulted in obvious failure. Today, people live religiously by what they read in diet books and fashion magazines, or by the information they hear on TV and from friends at a bar, the gym, at school; from colleagues at the office and even from family members. It often seems that everyone has a different answer, a new plan, a diet that can't miss, but all the while more and more people continue to grow ever so obese and become sick. People emphatically shout out the reasons from every direction, a scenario reminiscent of an early morning tuna auction at the fish market in the heart of Tokyo. It's the calories. No, it's the fats. The carbs. Too much time at the computer Hey, you better get out and exercise. Take vitamin B-12. It's in your genes. Did I hear genes? Going once, going twice ... SOLD! In fact, you've probably found yourself sold on every one of these facades at one time or another while still hoping that the scientific community will someday find the answer to the question that consumes you. Maybe they'll come up with something as simple as . . . a pill.

But then you look at dad, uncle Joey, mom, your sister Catalina … and you say to yourself, *"Why couldn't I have been born into a pool of skinny genes? Of all the things I could have inherited, it had to be the genes that make me fat."*

Many of you may have adhered to every new restrictive diet on the planet, taken every supplement, swallowed every diet pill and devoured the concept of low calorie, low fat diets, "healthy" hydrogenated fats and the high protein craze; only to find out later that these ideas were downright dangerous and have only brought you new health problems. At the same time you continue to wrestle with your weight issues and prepare to move on to the next promising diet. Sound familiar? The Yogurt Diet – which is, in essence, a lifestyle – will teach you how to put all these problems behind you once and for all, and you will learn why much of what you have previously believed about losing weight is mostly irrelevant.

Unfortunately, most of the popular diet recommendations of the past few decades are flawed and eventually make the dieter crash. Perhaps that's even where the term "crash diet" comes from? These diets are designed to keep you looking in the opposite direction instead of looking straight ahead, so you can't really get a clear picture of why you have an ongoing weight problem. It is, however, precisely this kind of thinking and longtime eating patterns that continue keeping so many people overweight. It's time that we finally face reality and begin looking for real answers. Up to now we have been putting our attention in all the wrong places.

The Yogurt Diet will give you the answers you need so that you take back control of your life. This is a lifestyle designed to keep you looking ahead so that you can get to your final destination safely, with grace and in a timely manner, while achieving your ideal weight and regaining radiant health. You will learn the real reasons why people become overweight and why that weight can be so difficult to lose. But take heart; there is hope. You've got to begin by realizing that your weight problem is not totally dictated by your genes and, as scientists are beginning to discover, it may also have less to do with the number of calories you eat, or even the time spent sitting at your desk in front of the computer than previously thought. The answers are straight ahead, so always keep looking forward. If you don't, you just might crash.

Your Relationship With Food

The relationship you have with food is a huge barometer of your eventual weight. *What* you eat, *when* you eat, *why* you eat and, *who* you eat with often determines whether you'll always be battling those extra pounds. The alternative is making peace with yourself and embracing both food and your whole being so you can begin creating a healthy relationship with something that's so essential for life – the nutrients you put in your body. Do you turn to food – the unhealthy kinds – whenever something goes wrong in your life? Is every emotional moment also an excuse to eat? If this is you, the reason is partly because of your history and longtime relationship with certain foods that you crave, such as apple pie with vanilla ice cream before going to bed each night.

Stop for a moment and think about your upbringing. What were you usually fed for breakfast, lunch and dinner? Was mealtime a family affair where everyone would partake in the preparation and serving, or did family members just wait to be called to the table? Were dinners mostly comprised of fast food, take out or frozen TV dinners, topped off with a finishing touch of double fudge chocolate macadamia nut cake? Or were dinners from your childhood a mix of happy family gatherings, a fresh fair of vegetables, rack of lamb in red wine jus and fresh baked bread, followed by fruit and creamy yogurt for dessert?

Behavior can accurately be called the "silent gene." The behavior you have around food is usually a product of what you have witnessed as a child from your parents, grandparents, siblings and society in general. That's why it's so important to remember how your family behaved around food when you were growing up. Because it is that same behavior you learned from your parents that is probably influencing your relationship with food today. To get a better idea, just take a moment and ask yourself some questions. Was your mom always on a diet? Did she restrict her food intake for a while, only to end up binging on all the wrong foods? Were fresh vegetables and fruits not a staple in your childhood diet? Did you constantly hear adults complain about their weight? Did anyone ever tell you that one day your body would look just like your mom's or dad's? All these questions and more lead to finding out what type of relationship you created with food from a very early age. Believe it or not, many answers lie hidden underneath these simple questions, and they can reveal one of the definitive reasons for the obesity epidemic as well as the outbreak of disease in our modern world. In fact, until you change your relationship with food you simply will not be able to put your battles with weight behind you.

I grew up on a farm outside the city of Madrid, in Spain. Dad was a fanatic about great food and always took care that the best of the best was at our table, while mom possessed the grace and magic in her fingers to prepare the most luscious dishes. The kitchen was always bursting with laughter, great stories and unforgettable aromas and flavors that still linger in my mind when I'm cooking my own recipes today. Needless to say, the kitchen was the most popular room in our home. Each season dad grew every vegetable imaginable that the region's weather and soil would permit. Fruit trees were scattered throughout, painting the landscape with magical colors when they bloomed. In the summer we had succulent peaches of every kind, the sweetest strawberries, juicy heirloom tomatoes, cucumbers, zucchini, carrots, eggplant, lettuce … I could go on forever. As the season turned and the chill in the air covered the early morning with frost, the vines would burst with grapes, the apple trees weighed down heavy with fruit, pomegranates, almonds and other delicious fresh foods were available in abundance. If we wanted an omelet, we'd run to the chicken house for fresh eggs. I'll never forget the feeling when entering the dark room and my small hands would touch the coops ever so carefully, looking to be warmly surprised by a newly laid egg!

It was like having a grocery store in your own back yard. In fact, sometimes we would play at just that. My oldest sister, Monica, who always had a flair for business, was the storeowner, while my brothers and I the loyal customers. With a rattan basket over our shoulder and the outmost determination to find just that perfect tomato that looked better than the rest, we would head to the garden and pick our favorite fruits, herbs and vegetables before running back to the kitchen. As we did our homework around the big wooden kitchen table the mix of aromas in the air teased our senses and we patiently waited for the feast that was to take place every night when dad arrived home.

This is how my passion for cooking and eating great food began and where I took my very first steps in the kitchen on my way to becoming a chef. Not surprisingly, these are also my earliest memories of food and the associations that go with it – happiness, love, warmth, comfort, feast, family, friends, earthiness, fun, passion and magic. And this continues to be what I carry in my heart when I cook and when I eat. It's also what I've always known food to be – fresh and seasonal produce picked just at the right time and eaten immediately, cooked by the loving hands which took care of me with delightful dishes throughout the earliest years of my life. When I eat today it is with the utmost pleasure and appreciation of the wonderful foods that are shared with friends, family and anyone I cook for or cooks for me. When you invest yourself in preparing food, you begin to appreciate the time and effort that goes into this endeavor and you become a conscious eater. What this means is that calories, fat and carbohydrates become a silly thing of the past. The conscious eater has more pressing concerns. Where did the ingredients come from? Are they the best quality? Who cooked the food, a person or a machine? Are these wholesome ingredients? Are the foods I'm about to eat processed or natural? Are the foods I'm eating promoting health or potentially causing disease within my body? These are some of the questions that always run through the mind of the conscious eater.

If you focus on changing learned behavior from your past you have already won half the battle. Begin exchanging packaged foods for wholesome ones, such as fruits and vegetables, grains and hormone-free animal proteins. Buying unpackaged foods not only saves money, but it also has a great impact on the planet because resources are not being wasted on unnecessary packaging. Better yet, if you have access to a farmer's market start making it a habit to buy most of your fruits and vegetables there. This helps support local farmers and conscientious farming practices. And then, of course, you'll have the singular pleasure of strolling down the stands under a sunny sky and looking for that perfect butternut squash to make a nourishing soup that fills up your home with the subtlety of autumn spices.

This may sound like a daunting task at first. But it's all about making changes one step at a time. To get into the swing of things, you can begin by cooking the easy and delicious recipes of the Yogurt Diet. Not only will you see pounds start to melt away, you'll also begin to create a healthy relationship with food and become a conscious eater, leaving behind the frightened eater who is constantly worrying about calories, carbohydrates and fats while sabotaging the right to enjoy the many pleasures of eating delicious and nurturing foods.

What Went Wrong

Going back in history you'll find that aside from war and cataclysmic events such as earthquakes and tornados, death was almost always caused by malnutrition and contagious disease, leading to epidemics and pandemics. The most frequent causes were a deficient food supply, poor hygiene and a lack of knowledge. Until the twentieth century arrived, people rarely died from obesity, heart disease, cancer, diabetes, and other illnesses that are, in the worst sense, a creation of modern lifestyle. It's almost certain that diseases such as cancer, obesity, ADD, food intolerances, diabetes, osteoporosis and heart disease have increased dramatically in the past fifty years. This obviously begs the question about the changes that have taken place in modernized countries over the past few decades and what they have really done.

It's easy to simplify the problems, to blame them on poor eating habits and a sedentary lifestyle, but it's really more complicated than that. As you will learn, every single one of modern life's diseases, such as obesity, diabetes and even colon cancer, are all connected in one way or another to one thing and one thing only – the change of *bacterial flora* in your digestive tract. That's right; the trillions of healthy bacteria that should be living inside everyone's digestive tract have been suffering a massive eviction in many of us since the last century. Believe it or not, one of the main causes is the advance of modern medicine (e.g. antibiotics); another is the foods we eat, as well as the old standby of stress. All these factors can contribute to the massacre of the healthy organisms in our digestive tract.

The body is, without doubt, a synergistic organism in which everything is connected and working together. But if one thing goes wrong, the result can be a domino effect that can topple even the healthiest person. At the apex of this cascading downward spiral is your diet. The foods you eat will determine your ultimate health and weight. The reason — you guessed it — is the enormous influence your diet has on your gut flora. In many cases, it is the correct balance of friendly bacteria in the GI tract that acts as the mediator to the many chemical reactions that take place in your body and are needed for optimum health and ideal weight.

Unfortunately, throughout the years, most of the efforts to solve the mystery of obesity and those extra stubborn pounds have been focused on the obvious culprits — proteins, fats, carbohydrates and the lack of exercise — when in reality, a main focus of attention should have been on the gut flora that colonize the digestive tract, which is our immune system's first line of defense.

It's ironic, but if you look at many of the small villages around the world, the inhabitants have known instinctively for centuries how to prevent disease while promoting life by consuming plenty of fermented milk products in their daily diets. It is only in modern society – despite all the wonderful scientific advances – that we have lost the knowledge our ancestors provided and, by living in the fast-paced present, have forgotten entirely about our past. Yet, as is often the case, looking back at our heritage may hold the key to finding the necessary answers to regaining our health without drugs and expensive medical treatments.

What is the Real Reason People Become Fat?

Suppose, like so many people today, you live in the so-called fast lane. Among other things, there's no time for real grocery shopping, let alone time to cook. The food industry foresaw this dilemma and took steps to solve the problem by inventing new ways to make your life easier. The trouble is that you're now compelled to buy ready-made foods that allegedly take care of the eating problem. That's right, the *eating problem!* There's only one thing wrong with this philosophy. Eating shouldn't be a problem. On the contrary, it is one of life's greatest pleasures, not to mention an absolute necessity. But for whatever reason, many people today have come to the conclusion that it is a problem. Here's why.

To begin with, many people would prefer to be doing something else rather than taking the time to prepare a nourishing meal that can be truly enjoyed and savored. Secondly, somewhere along the way we've been led to believe that food is all the same, and thus it's simply excess calories from food that is the real cause of the obesity epidemic. So we shy away from food in general, often demonizing this essential means of sustenance in our lives. Ironically, this set of beliefs can all be traced back to the relationship you have created with food from your personal experiences, and from information relayed to you by your parents, siblings, friends, books, magazines, TV, co-workers and other so called experts. Unfortunately, much of this information is just plain wrong — inaccurate, exaggerated and unbalanced — and really serves little purpose if what you're looking for is to achieve lifetime results. So all this must change.

Remember, wholesome foods ingested into a balanced body cannot make you fat. They simply can't! Wholesome foods keep both body and mind working at their best, and make sure the body is fit and healthy. But the operative word here is **balance**.

Now let's take a look at some of the biggest offenders and major contributors to both the obesity epidemic and the spread of so many modern diseases. I think you'll be happy to learn that none of these negative contributors can be classified as "real" foods. For example, you will not see any negative connotations associated with the words calories, carbohydrates and fats anywhere in this book. To the contrary, I strongly support these three often demonized words and for a very simple reason. We all need these nutrients in our bodies to be thin and healthy. It's that simple. Here's why.

Calories are energy, and who among us doesn't want or need energy? An energetic person is far more appealing and sexy than a lethargic one. As for carbohydrates, they are not only delicious, but also provide many necessary vitamins and minerals that contribute to sustaining a healthy body, as well as being an essential force to metabolize those oh-so-fearsome calories. In addition, carbs are a great source of all-important fiber. Healthy fats — such as those found in extra virgin olive oil, cold pressed coconut oil and butter, nuts, eggs, milk products and meats derived from naturally raised animals, and fish to name a few — are essential for a brilliantly working mind, prevent cardiovascular disease and maintain youthful looking skin, among many other functions.

Hopefully, as you read on, you will begin to make changes — mentally at first — in the relationship you have with food and begin to accept the fact that food is not your enemy, but rather an important and friendly ally. You'll also be amazed when you finally realize how much misinformation about food you've assimilated from so many different sources over the years, and then you'll be pleasantly surprised to learn that the weight problems afflicting our society today may have very little to do with food. Whenever I talk about food, I always mean wholesome foods – not something that is processed, denatured, wrapped, canned, machine made, precooked and overcooked, and pasteurized. These are food "items," not food in the true meaning of the word.

According to the dictionary, food must provide nutrients, growth, nourishment and energy, as well as stimulate the mind and soul. If what you're eating does not meet these requirements, then it shouldn't be considered food. The problem today is that so many of us are eating *food items* in the guise of real food. Real food, plain and simple, plays no part in the obesity and disease epidemics that continue to assault our society. Food is food, produce that comes from the land right into your loving hands, then into the kitchen and finally to your table. This is the ONLY processing food needs — the love and passion from your hands and heat from the stove.

Unfortunately, this simple maxim rarely exists today. It is all the extras added to our food before it reaches us, coupled with our modern and hectic lifestyles that are the guilty parties when it comes to promoting weight gain and disease. A sampling of these "extras" include chlorinated water, high fructose corn syrup, sugar, highly processed carbohydrates and proteins, hydrogenated oils, antibiotics as well as other drugs, animal hormones and excess alcohol. These are some of the offenders that promote weight gain. Not food! And the reason these are to blame for our twenty-first century health problems is because they all contribute to the death of our good old friends, the *healthy* gut flora. The biggest threat to your well-being from these dangerous offenders is in the destruction and starvation of the healthy bacteria as they cross your digestive tract, the place where trillions of healthy micro-organisms make their home and whose survival depends so much on what you consciously eat everyday. New evidence is beginning to suggest that the lack of a healthy fauna of bacteria in the digestive track may be the biggest contributor to the obesity epidemic we face today.

Fortunately, the battle is not yet lost. Yogurt, a miraculous food, is loaded with nutrients that not only nourish the body but also replenishes the depleted gut flora in the intestines with plenty of probiotic bacteria. Thus the Yogurt Diet is designed to work on several levels and has a dual purpose. First, the Yogurt Diet is healthy and wholesome in itself because it is based on traditionally safe world diets and cuisines. Second, its purpose is to re-establish bacterial colonies in the digestive tract so that the all-important job of bringing balance back into your body can be accomplished. As this happens, you'll also find the pounds melting away and, at the same time, witness your health flourishing. In fact, once you've finished reading this chapter my guess is you'll not only be convinced that food is not the enemy, but you will embrace the Yogurt Diet without hesitation.

Interestingly, all the offenders I will be discussing in the following pages have crept, slowly and silently, into our lives during the twentieth century, with most of them gaining widespread acceptance sometime after World War II. And that is precisely the point in time that we can pinpoint the beginnings of the obesity epidemic and the increased incidents of cancer, heart disease and other ailments. A coincidence? Read on and be the judge.

The Six Ruthless Offenders

The following is a list of things the conscious eater should avoid. These items are the biggest promoters of weight gain and loss of health in our lives today. Here, in detail, is what these modern day offenders can do to you if taken into your body on a regular basis.

1. Chlorinated Water: A "Safer" Water Supply

It was in 1904 when someone first got the bright idea to chlorinate the drinking water. Jersey City, New Jersey, was the first American city to have a chlorinated reservoir. The purpose was noble, to stop the spread of disease caused by contaminated waters. But it was really not until the 1940's that chlorination became widespread throughout the United States.

In its purest form, water from uncontaminated natural resources contains living organisms as well as minerals that are beneficial to all living things, including humans. In an industrialized world, however, the available water supply is far from pure. Rather, it is contaminated with many harmful organisms that pose a serious health risk to humans. Therefore, preventative measures must be put in place. Chlorination of water has been the choice to disinfect water for more than a century. It is a great bacterial killer, keeping certain harmful organisms at bay and preventing disease and death to humans. That's great. Unfortunately, there's also a downside. Just as chlorine kills harmful bacteria in water, it also kills the good bacteria in the digestive tract when you drink it. As the chlorine present in water passes throughout the GI tract it causes the flora in the intestines to die off and that's when bad things begin to happen. This leaves the door open for harmful organisms to proliferate in areas of your body where good bacteria normally live. Then, slowly, your immune system begins to fail and with it your health.

Researchers have a wealth of evidence that among people who drink chlorinated water the chances of contracting heart disease, Hodgkin's disease and a variety of cancers, including cancer of the colon, bladder, gastrointestinal tract, esophagus and breast all become greater. The risk is over 40 percent more prevalent than for those who don't drink chlorinated waters.

Ironically, chlorination was put in place to kill harmful bacteria and to prevent certain deadly diseases. This was successful and has certainly saved many lives. But the same chlorination that prevents disease from contaminated waters also kills the good bacteria present in your digestive tract, causing an increase in other diseases that today are also responsible for ending lives.

What can you do if your water supply is chlorinated? First, begin drinking bottled water. Secondly, buy a water filter for your home. You can refill bottles and keep them in the refrigerator. Also, use cool running filtered water to clean your vegetables. There's no need to use any special soaps to clean fruits and vegetables. A few wonderful water filters exist in the market today to extract chlorine and other poisonous substances from water. These self-installed water filters are also quite affordable.

2. Antibiotics —The Irony of the Anti-Life Drug that Saves Lives

By definition alone, antibiotic means "against life," and is the antithesis of probiotic. That should tell you something immediately. An antibiotic is an agent used against living organisms to treat bacterial infections. However, antibiotics don't work against viral, fungal or other microbial infections. At the same time, they are quite possibly on the list of the top three most frequently prescribed medications, with more than 100 different types of antibiotics available today.

The over-prescribing of antibiotics is a terrifying fact. Just as antibiotics kill harmful bacteria, they also eradicate the healthful bacteria meant to live in your body to promote life. Antibiotics don't discriminate between good or bad bacteria. They simply kill all bacteria in their path. When you consume antibiotics to treat an infection, you're also creating a great imbalance within your body as a result of the extermination of your friendly bacterial gut flora. Remember, a healthy gut flora means a smooth-functioning immune system. Once the immune system is compromised, opportunistic organisms such as yeasts and a number of parasites — which aren't affected by antibiotics — can start reproducing uncontrollably and take over your digestive system. This, in turn, can cause symptoms such as diarrhea, negative reactions to milk and wheat, sugar cravings, vaginal yeast infections, acid reflux, gas, bloating, skin diseases, GI disorders, bad breath and hair loss, just to name a few negative side effects that occur over time from taking antibiotics.

Sadly, this is only the beginning, because if you don't take steps to reestablish the normal flora of probiotic bacteria in your digestive tract after having taken antibiotics, harmful organisms will spiral out of control and the consequences can soon result in obesity, cancer, diabetes, heart disease, hypertension, infertility, IBS, acne and so on. Sound familiar? Not surprisingly, these are some of the same diseases associated with the consumption of chlorinated water and they occur simply because chlorinated water and antibiotics have the same effect in your digestive tract. They both kill the friendly bacteria that nature put in place to protect the body from disease and maintain a healthy weight.

Antibiotics are one of the wonder drugs of the modern era that take care of one problem but create a new one. Only the progression on the back end is much slower and often goes unrecognized. The deterioration of one's health that occurs after taking antibiotics is often a slow process, which makes it difficult to connect the dots and prove the correlation between antibiotic intake, overall poor health and sudden weight gain. Maybe that's why it has taken so long before anyone recognized the link between antibiotic use and diminished health. But with more research being done, the evidence is becoming irrefutable.

Thanks to antibiotics, millions of lives have undoubtedly been saved over the past half-century. But sadly, these drugs have also become wildly available and are often over-prescribed by physicians who often don't consider the harmful side effects these drugs can promote. Doctors should really be more selective when prescribing antibiotics and each individual should choose carefully when to take them. However, if you find yourself in the position where you must take antibiotics, be sure to follow the Yogurt Diet during and after your antibiotic prescription. This will ensure that you rebuild your immune system by re-establishing your beneficial gut flora and pushing harmful organisms out of the way. If you develop the type of infection that requires antibiotics, it is a clear sign that your immune system has been compromised in the first place. Then the Yogurt Diet becomes even more of a necessity in order to prevent this situation from becoming repetitive.

One effective way to combat microbial infections is …with yogurt. Yes, yogurt with its probiotic bacteria replenishes the body's gut flora that the immune system needs to fight off pathogens. LAB create an acidic environment in parts of the GI tract, which promotes a hostile environment where harmful organisms cannot survive. LAB will also compete with and displace the harmful bacteria or yeasts. The re-establishment of good bacteria is a preventative measure that builds your immune system and ensures that you remain healthy. It is only when your bacterial flora suffers and allows harmful organisms to take over that you become susceptible to various infections that require you to take antibiotics. This can become a vicious cycle.

Many people who take antibiotics never fully regain their health. By not re-establishing a balanced gut flora, they continue to experience a downward spiral of symptoms that leads to "feeling bad all over." Then guess what? In many cases more antibiotics will be prescribed and, sooner or later, many could end up being diagnosed with a disease that has a frightening name. What, then, is the solution? Eat yogurt; eat it often and follow the delicious Yogurt Diet to regain balance. This will not only help re-establish your healthy flora, it will also rebuild a strong immune system, ensuring you don't get sick again. In fact, it should become standard care for doctors to prescribe probiotic yogurt during and after a prescription of antibiotics.

Yet there is a better way. Prevention. That's the real key and my mantra. Prevent, prevent, prevent . . . with yogurt and a wholesome diet.

More Bad News About Antibiotics

Another disconcerting fact about antibiotics is that even when you choose not to take them, you may still be consuming them indirectly if the animal products you eat don't come from sustainable farming practices. Many commercially farmed animals are fed antibiotics in their daily diets for two reasons. One is to prevent disease, even if there is no sign of disease, and the second is to fatten up animals with a class of antibiotics called GPA's (growth-promoting antibiotics). How very interesting, an antibiotic fed to animals to make them fat. That alone should tell you something about the damage antibiotics can do and the way it can affect your weight. Chose to consume milk products, meats, eggs and chicken from animals that have not been administered antibiotics and growth hormones. The residue of antibiotics in animal foods can have the same harmful effects in your body when passing through your intestinal tract during digestion — contributing to the depletion of your healthy gut flora and resulting in fattening you up. Fortunately, the food industry is working hard to establish measures and controls in which antibiotic residue from animal products are removed from our food supply. It can't happen too soon.

3. Sugar and High Fructose Corn Syrup — The Silent Killer

What we commonly know as table sugar is derived from cane. It is basically sucrose, which is a disaccharide, meaning that it has two simple sugar molecules attached together. They are equal parts glucose and fructose. During digestion in the stomach and in the small intestine, sucrose is broken down into fructose and glucose by the enzyme *sucrase*. This process is called inversion, and it is the method in which the body regulates the rate of sucrose breakdown. Without this mechanism in place, the body has less control over the rate of sugar absorption into the bloodstream, so this is a very good thing.

In the case of high fructose corn syrup (HFCS), however, the sugar molecules glucose and fructose are not attached together. Instead, the sugars are "free" and more readily available to be absorbed very quickly into the body. Also, the percentage of fructose to glucose is up to nine times higher, making the ratio about 90 percent fructose and 10 percent glucose. Glucose is metabolized in every cell of the body, whereas fructose must always be metabolized by the liver first, putting a real burden in this organ and not allowing the pancreas to release insulin, a process that can induce insulin resistance. If this abuse of over consumption of fructose continues for a long period of time, inflammation of the liver occurs, resulting in a fatty liver and cirrhosis. Glucose and fructose are both metabolized in the liver, which then converts sugars into triglycerides. This process leads to an excess of lipids (fats) in the body, which then can lead to obesity and cardiovascular disease.

Over consumption of sugar (sucrose) can be harmful to your health and you should limit its intake. However, many studies have concluded that the real danger lies in high fructose corn syrup because of the reasons stated above and in the way it interferes with many of the body's natural chemical reactions in the metabolism of foods. Consumed over a long period of time, high fructose corn syrup will encourage obesity and diabetes, as well as it hampers the body's use of magnesium, chromium and copper, three minerals that are essential for the heart and immune system to function properly.

Unfortunately, both of these ingredients — high fructose corn syrup and sugar — are present in almost every pre-made and packaged food on the shelves of supermarkets and in nearly all fast foods. And because of the way so many Americans eat today, much too much of these ingredients are making their way into the body and the digestive tract.

The United States is the biggest grower of corn in the world and the largest producer of its byproducts, including high fructose corn syrup. In 1982, a system was put in place by the U.S. government for price supports of imports, and sugar was struck particularly hard with high U.S. import quotas and tariffs. It made the price of sugar in the United States inordinately expensive and nearly twice what the rest of the world pays. The American food industry, in an attempt to keep product prices low, immediately switched to high-fructose corn syrup, which had been introduced in the United States commercially in the 1970's. HFCS rapidly became a sugar substitute in the vast majority of American processed foods and soft drinks after 1982, making corn syrup the sweetener of choice and one of the main food preservatives in the industry. Today, HFCS is found in cereals, soft drinks, fast foods, fruit juices, pasta sauces, condiments, beer, bacon, select "health products," frozen foods, flavored yogurts, breads, bakery goods ... and many, many other common processed foods.

At the same time, the American government has programs in place, which contribute to the low cost of corn with subsidies designed to lure farmers into producing more. Corn is not a vegetable, but rather a grain, which yields many uses and almost no waste. Among other things, corn's many uses include human and animal feed, corn oil, as a sweetener and preservative in the form of high fructose syrup and, more recently, even as bio fuel.

Calories and Corn

Concerned about calories? Just as a side note, you may want to know that corn is an excellent energy source. Because it yields so much more energy than any other grain, corn is the grain of choice by farmers as feed for their animal stock in order to fatten them up. Great steak houses serve only meat from animals that have been fed corn. Why? Because the high caloric diet, mostly form sugars in corn, yields an extremely high content of fat in the meat, and that makes it more flavorful than a lean piece of meat from a grass fed animal.

Understandably, many international food corporations continue to use sugar, but due to its high price in the United States these same corporations use only high fructose corn syrup for food and beverage products sold in the U.S. Comparing the increased consumption of HFCS and the rise of obesity in America since the 1980's, there seems to be a definite correlation. The Center for Disease Control has documented this exorbitant increase of obesity in the population over the past 30 years, the same period during which the American food industry converted from sugar to HFCS. Can we conclude that this is simply a coincidence? We could, but I would dare to argue that the trend in the increased use of high fructose corn syrup may yet be one more cause in the rise of obesity and disease over the past few decades.

Not surprisingly, high fructose corn syrup also kills your intestinal flora and provides a source of energy for fungi, such as Candida. Individuals who eat a lot of processed foods also, by default, eat a diet that is full of sugar and corn syrup, but one devoid of wholesome, nutrient rich foods. This lifestyle — and it is often a self-perpetuating one — starves the bacteria in the intestinal tract and gives rise to the harmful organisms that feed off sugars, organisms that would ordinarily mingle in minor numbers among the rest of the dominant, healthy flora. Pathogens love sweet foods and all other simple sugars. When you eat a diet rich in these types of foods, the bad guys spread and take over by displacing the fauna of probiotics that normally live in a healthy intestinal tract. And if harmful organisms conquer your digestive tract, guess what happens next? You experience cravings for more of the same foods that are full of high fructose corn syrup, sugar and processed carbs, allowing the harmful organisms to proliferate even more.

Before long, you become literally addicted to the same foods. And when this addiction leads you to overeat, the extra calories will result in more weight gain. By this time you're robbing your body of nutrients and causing pathogenic organisms to ultimately drive you to the over-consumption of offending foods so that they can continue their proliferation. As you might have guessed, this pattern of eating will continue as part of a vicious cycle. More weight gain is inevitable unless you start making changes in your life by avoiding antibiotics, foods that contain sugar and high fructose corn syrup, processed foods and pasteurized fruit juices. When you reach the point at which your body is in a state of imbalance, all the calorie counting and willpower will be of little help if you're putting these wrong foods in your body regularly. To make your weight loss efforts count and become permanent you must first create harmony and balance by eating a variety of healthy foods and consuming yogurt daily.

The hidden danger of processed fruit juices is yet another modern day food tragedy. Most people are convinced that they're making a "healthy" choice when they chose to drink bottled fruit juice over a soda. However, in essence, the two are very similar. Let me explain. Fruits are super foods and you should eat them every day. They are not only delicious; they're also rich in many vitamins, minerals, antioxidants, fiber, carbohydrates and other beneficial compounds. But fruits are complex individuals with nothing simple about them. The sugar in fruits is fructose, and this sugar is simply one element among the many pieces of the fruit puzzle.

Here's where the problem begins. When fruits are broken apart, separated from their elements and pasteurized, as it's the case with packaged fruit juices, their complexity suffers and nutrients are lost, leaving behind pure sugar in the form of fructose. During pasteurization, fructose is heated to high temperatures, which makes it become concentrated and denatured. Sadly, this is how a good thing loses its reputation and begins to get the bad rap that fruits are getting these days with the popularized "low carb" diets. Fruits are some of the healthiest and yummiest foods on the planet. Try blending bananas with yogurt and crushed pecans. I can't begin to explain what a delicious snack this makes. And if you want to enjoy a cold glass of orange juice make it at home, fresh squeezed. A citric juice maker may be the most affordable luxury you will ever own. Once you taste real fresh squeezed juice, you'll never want to have anything else. In future chapters you will learn why you should always combine fruits with yogurt. It makes all the difference when you're trying to lose weight. This is a little Yogurt Diet secret…shhhhh.

More on High Fructose Corn Syrup

In the European Union, the production of high fructose corn syrup (HFCS), known as isoglucose, is limited under a sugar regime put in place since 1977. Only three percent of the total production of sugar is allowed to come from corn syrup. Because of this law, sugar is still the sweetener of choice in Europe, where the obesity problem is obviously not as acute as in the United States. North Americans consume 44.1 pounds of high fructose corn syrup per person per year, in addition to 72.8 pounds of refined sugar

4. Stress

How many times have you heard someone say, perhaps even your doctor, "If you don't stop worrying so much and stressing out, you're going to make yourself sick?" When I was a kid I can remember adults saying, "Don't stress out, or you'll give yourself an ulcer." I once asked mom what an ulcer was and she told me that an ulcer is a wound in the stomach. As a child the possibility of causing an internal wound from being angry and sad seemed highly impossible. It didn't make sense. But as I found out later, ulcers are caused by an overgrowth of certain harmful bacteria. This malicious intruder goes by the name of Helicobacter pylori. Now, of course, it makes perfect sense. Stress can be a killer. Literally. During episodes of anger and stressful times, the stomach produces excess acids, which not only burn the lining of the digestive tract, but also kill the good bacteria that line the mucus walls. Ulcers, then, are sores on the lining of the digestive tract. The most common ulcer is located in the duodenum. Another type of ulcer located in the stomach is called a gastric ulcer, and result in the ailment known as gastritis. But regardless of the name and location, all ulcers are caused by a bacterial infection.

Scientific studies have produced strong evidence equating anger related stress with the alteration of the gut flora in the digestive tract. Not surprisingly, many modern diseases are intestine-related, from Irritable Bowl Syndrome (IBS); to Inflammatory Bowl Disease (IBD), which includes ulcerative colitis and Crohn's disease; to colon cancer; metabolic syndrome; acid reflux and ulcers, to name a few. In each case, we must question if the causes are not due to an imbalance of the microbiota in the digestive tract and an impaired mucosal barrier of the GI tract, obviously caused by the absence of good bacteria and its replacement by pathogenic organisms.

Studies also show that anger, stress, fright and depression produce a distinct gut flora change upon the colon and upper digestive tract, due to the over production of two hormones, adrenalin and gastrin. Under these circumstances your body is in fight-or-flight response, which means that when the body perceives threat and danger many physiological changes begin to take place, one of them being the way food passes through your digestive tract. The changes include intestinal motility (movement of food), intestinal blood flow, gastric and colonic secretions, nutrient absorption, and bile absorption and secretion. These are exactly the same changes known to produce gastric and duodenal ulcers. If you suffer from colitis, IBS or ulcers, you now have the insight to what may very well be causing your symptoms.

But take heart, there is something you can do to alleviate your condition and even perhaps resolve the problem, and that is embracing the Yogurt Diet. There are two rules you must follow in order to achieve this goal. One, you need to cleanse your system of toxins and harmful organisms and, two; your healthy gut flora must be reintroduced with the help of probiotic yogurt. These two steps will bring your body back into harmony and you will regain your health.

This remedy, although simple, is a lot more than just wishful thinking. A number of scientists have conducted studies to prove that fer-

Bacteria and Ulcers

Australian scientists Barry J. Marshal and J. Robin Warren were the two brilliant minds that first recognized that ulcers are caused by an infectious growth of the bacteria Helicobacter pylori. This idea met much resistance at first, as the medical community once firmly believed that ulcers were a chronic disease without a cure. The two persevered, though it finally took the courage of Barry J. Marshal to ingest a culture of the harmful bacteria, H. pylori, and make himself sick with an ulcer to prove their theory. In 2005 they both shared the Nobel Prize for this wonderful discovery!

mented milk products, such as yogurt, can displace the harmful bacteria that cause ulcers by replacing the damaged areas with beneficial organisms to promote healing. Conventional antibiotic treatment, usually the choice of doctors to treat this condition, has been proven unnecessary to treat ulcers and achieve total recovery. Studies show, in fact, that the only remedy needed to get patients back to health was simply good, old-fashioned yogurt.

Additional evidence points at chronic stress and early traumas in life as a reason for the change of gut physiology and the failing of various important bodily functions. The good news, however, is that several reliable studies have now concluded that ingesting live probiotic bacteria found in yogurt during stressful times can reduce these problems before they spiral out of control, and can stop harmful organisms in their tracks. The probiotic bacteria in yogurt strengthen the mucosal barrier in the digestive tract and prevent the invasion of disease causing bacteria, parasites and allergens.

Another year long study confirmed that under a constant anger/stress situation, dramatic changes took place in the gut of subjects under examination in just ten days. Among the symptoms documented were diarrhea, weight fluctuations, and harmful species of microorganisms colonizing and penetrating into the intestinal protective barrier, resulting in inflammation. This is a dangerous and vicious cycle that can be avoided if you vigilantly follow a wholesome diet and eat plenty of yogurt during times of stress. Chronic stress leads to the depletion of the first intestinal line of defense, the gut flora. This, in turn, gives room for harmful bacteria to take over by attaching themselves and penetrating through the protective mucosal barrier of the GI tract, the second line of defense. When this happens, the result is inflammation, followed by pain, which in itself leads to more chronic stress.

When you're stressed out it's very important to maintain a healthful diet, because any time the body is under constant pressure it quickly becomes psychologically and physically unbalanced. Many people also experience weight loss during stressful times. Conversely, as the cause of

Fight-Or-Flight Response

This is the body's response to perceived threat or danger, a mechanism that enables us to physically fight or run away when faced with danger. But in our modern lives, often filled with chronic stress, this response can be erroneously activated when dealing with traffic, money problems, abusive relationships, etc. When the perceived threat is gone, systems are designed to return back to normal function via the relaxation response. Unfortunately, in our stressful society this often doesn't happen and the constant stress levels can cause damage to all systems in the body, while also contributing to the depletion of the healthy gut flora. Therefore, unless you correct the situation with stress management and diet, both aimed to replenish your gastrointestinal flora, the damage can become chronic and develop into the many diseases that are so prevalent today.

your stress either wanes or becomes magnified, sugar cravings caused by the overgrowth of pathogenic organisms lead to overeating and weight gain. This is one explanation of why we can easily put on a few pounds during and even after stressful times. Research shows, however, that consumption of certain types of beneficial bacteria while under stress prevents the adherence and penetration of harmful organisms into the protective barriers of the intestines.

Have you also ever wondered why, during times of stress, you get sick easily? The reason is simple. When your healthy gut flora is displaced, your immune system — your third line of defense — suffers and becomes vulnerable for a takeover by pathogenic bacteria, yeast and viruses, thus you become more susceptible to the common cold or flu. People in this situation will often go to the doctor and come home with a prescription for antibiotics. This just perpetuates the situation, adding even further imbalance to your body. Is everything beginning to make sense? By now, the best recourse should be obvious. During stressful times, how about instead of taking a "chill pill," you add probiotic yogurt to your diet three times a day?

5. Lack of Sleep

Stress often has yet another byproduct, a lack of sleep. The two go together because they invariably create a winning team for disaster. Good sleep is a fundamental part of good health. In fact, you can make a case that both sleeping and eating are the two more important essentials for life.

If someone in Spain wants to gain weight the age old formula to make it happen is skipping siesta. During that glorious time that we have in Spain, it is recommended that instead of taking the customary little nap you simply lie down but not fall asleep. The key here is not falling asleep. If you fall asleep it doesn't count. I remember a very thin young lady, Rosa, from my hometown who wanted to gain weight for her wedding day. The local doctor suggested she deprive herself of sleep. Within just a couple of months she gained enough weight that she had to resize her wedding dress!

This may sound like a funny story, at best, if not far fetched. But a group of researchers have found that this phenomenon may be due to biological mechanisms, and they question whether too much emphasis has been put on diet and lack of exercise when, in fact, all you may really need is a good night's sleep. Studies say that people who sleep less are more likely to have a weight problem. Or maybe it works the other way? Do overweight people have a problem falling asleep? This can certainly create yet another vicious cycle that can be difficult to break, and lead to another stressful situation.

The body is actually going through a detoxification process during all hours of the day, both when you're awake and sleeping. But it is during your restful zzzz's that this process goes into full swing. If the body is deprived of this essential cleansing, it begins to accumulate toxins.

But being the amazingly designed machine it is, the body has a mechanism to protect itself from the excess toxins it cannot shed and which can harm your health. These toxic substances are dutifully transported to fat cells, where the lipids in the cell walls act as an insulating barrier to stop pathogens from escaping into your blood stream and then into various organs in the body. As more toxins are stored, the fat cells grow larger, and you know what that means. The inflammation of fat cells results in exactly what you probably expect . . . obvious accumulation of fat.

The National Institute of Health is so supportive of this plausible new theory that it is increasing its resources to continue investigating what is still considered an enigma. While research is really just beginning, what I do know for certain is that Rosa turned her languished silhouette into a voluptuous figure just by skipping siesta.

If your desire is to lose weight, join a yoga class, practice meditation, and learn to deal with problems that arise in your life with grace and less stress. Go to bed early with a warm cup of chamomile tea by your bedside, relax and think beautiful thoughts with your eyes closed. Imagine all the amazing things you could do if you woke up every morning rested and fully energized. You would be as light as a dandelion floating in the wind, not just in mind, but in body as well.

6. Poor Diet

I hope you saw this one coming.

What you eat and drink has a great impact not only on your weight, but also on your health. When you eat sugar laden, processed and overcooked foods without an abundance of vitamins, minerals, amino acids, fatty acids, antioxidants, enzymes and live organisms, you are eating, in the very true sense of the word, dead foods. These foods add no life-promoting benefits to your body, except for bulk in your belly and what we know as empty calories. These types of foods may give you a quick boost of energy, but very little of anything else. Furthermore, your intestinal probiotic flora needs the same healthy foods as the rest of your body. If you starve them, they'll slowly but surely die off.

There are two ways in which nutrients and calories from the foods you eat are absorbed into your system. One is through the villi, the tiny, finger-like hairs lining the small intestine that normally allow the organ to absorb nutrients into the bloodstream, and the second is through the metabolic processes of probiotic bacteria in your colon. This is a sophisticated system put in place to extract every little healthy nutrient from the foods you eat, nutrients that are otherwise not accessible to enter your body through the small intestine. When you consume a diet full of simple sugars and highly processed foods, the majority of those foods are very easily absorbed by the small intestine, which leaves very few nutrients left to feed the gut flora in the colon. Subsequently, you starve the little friendly guys at the end of the food chain in your digestive tract — so important to maintain ideal weight and health — that they eventually die off.

Alcohol has been traditionally used as a sterilizer to kill bacteria. What makes you think, then, that it doesn't have same effect in your GI tract? Over-consumption of alcohol is another contributor to the depletion of your probiotic bacteria, which in turn also promotes the growth of harmful organisms — in particular dangerous yeasts — known to accelerate weight gain and loss of health. A glass of wine can only be beneficial when your body is in tip top shape, but when large quantities of alcohol are consumed repeatedly this will contribute to the death of the healthy flora in the digestive tract and the proliferation of harmful organisms. Invariably, this will lead to extra pounds on your mid-section and accumulation of pockets of fat in various parts of your body in the form of cellulite.

As you continue reading you will learn that old standards of counting calories, fats, points or carbs are effective only for a short period of time. These widely popularized and standard recommendations to promote weight loss are very short lived and generally excruciating experiences, as they're not permanent solutions to the weight battles. It is the quality of the foods rather than the amount you eat which will ultimately have the most impact on your weight and health. Processed foods, low fat, low carb, low cal, high protein, denatured packaged foods, excess consumption of alcohol, along with sugar, antibiotics, birth control pills, steroids, and other medications are the parts of your diet that are the real contributors to weight gain, because they cause the depletion of your healthy bacteria in the intestines. And by now you know what happens after that.

Now You Have the Facts

If you have been assaulting your body with chlorinated water, antibiotics, stress, lack of sleep, processed foods and alcohol, it is quite possible that you have created a huge imbalance in your bacterial ecosystem. When this occurs, all the systems in your body begin to shut down slowly — digestion becomes inefficient, a lack of enzymes occurs, your metabolism slows down, your immune response fails, hormones stop being produced, your body becomes toxic and you begin to suffer the consequences with disease and excessive weight gain.

At this point, no diet targeted simply to cut down caloric intake is going to help you lose weight and regain your health. And the last thing you need is more medication to make your body even more toxic and prone to disease. Instead, what you need is a great cleansing plan aimed to detoxify your body from pathogenic substances and polluting organisms. You need an eating plan that focuses on bringing balance back to your entire body. The Yogurt Diet was formulated to teach you how to bring harmony to every system of the body — by detoxifying and replenishing.

It will become absolutely clear how the body not only begins to accumulate weight when it's unbalanced, but how it also becomes diseased when you consume the wrong diet. In addition, you'll find out just what has always stopped you from losing weight and feeling absolutely fantastic. And finally, you will embrace food as a positive reinforcement in your life while throwing away the boring and taxing notion of counting calories, points, carbs, fats, and eating tasteless packaged foods.

Chapter Four

Here Come the Gut Bugs

Let me begin by asking if you, or anyone you know, suffer from the following ailments or disorders. Some of them have been mentioned before, but because of the nature of the material in this chapter, I think it's important to repeat them here. They are — in no special order — obesity, localized weight, diabetes, high cholesterol, skin disorders, celiac disease, lactose intolerance, chronic fatigue, gastric reflux, eating disorders, painful bloating and gas, hormonal imbalances, ADD, periodontal disease, bad breath, migraine headaches, infertility, impotence, auto-immune disorders, urinary tract infections, yeast infections, nail fungus, IBS, gastrointestinal ulcers, ulcerative colitis, Crohn's disease, polyps and cancer. This is a list that continues to grow. And if you live in the twenty-first century, you probably know people who have a number of these ailments and should count yourself lucky if you don't.

Believe it or not, these symptoms and disorders were, for the most part, quite rare some100 years ago. Today, however, they're all common maladies, especially among the populations of modern societies.

The Yogurt Diet was consciously formulated to provide answers to the increasing frequency of these diseases and ailments, and will give you a natural and simple way to become healthy again.

Growing up in Spain I never heard of anyone who suffered from any of these ills, children or adults. Rarely did I ever see an overweight man, woman or child, not in Spain and not when traveling throughout the Mediterranean region. Obesity, per se, simply didn't exist. But today, even from the tender childhood years when we're supposed to be the epitome of vitality, we must learn about diseases such as obesity, diabetes, allergies, food intolerances, ADD and ADHD. When we are old enough, we graduate with honors from these ailments, only to move on to bigger and "greater" complaints with more grown up names, such as high cholesterol, high blood pressure, heart attacks, infertility, arthritis, impotence, hypothyroid, cancer, and some other hair rising, toe curling scary diseases.

Weight gain and illness occur in the body due to an internal response that alerts us when something is out of balance. In other words, our bodies don't get sick without good reason. The entire body is a synergy, the total sum of all the parts involved. The immune system is your body's foundation to prevent and fight disease. At the forefront of the immune system is the well-trained army of healthy bacterial soldiers that line the mucus surfaces of many parts of the body, such as the walls of the intestinal tract, respiratory tract, the vagina and even the skin. We should literally be covered with bacteria that protect us. When an imbalance of healthy flora occurs in your immune system, it opens the door for a cascade-like effect, resulting in acute inflammation and eventually leading to chronic disease. Any of these aforementioned symptoms are a sure sign that your body is suffering from a serious imbalance. Instead of medicating the imbalance, it's important to get to the root cause, treat it and eradicate it by reestablishing harmony within your body.

Chronic inflammation of an organ or tissue can lead to disease. Again, this situation may arise when the probiotic bacterial flora in your digestive tract is depleted and harmful organisms see an opportunity to take over. With these pathogenic microbes in control, disease becomes more likely to occur. Once these malicious guys become established, your remaining good bacteria must work harder than ever to push invaders out, but it isn't easy.

Parasites

Parasites are harmful organisms that live inside or on another living organism, benefiting from the host for a prolonged time and causing damage. Most living things, including humans, have at least one parasite that feeds off them. Parasites are highly sophisticated creatures that are rather ruthless in their survival tactics. They can hide from the host's immune system so that they will not be identified and subsequently driven out, while at the same time continuing to impair the health of the host and exploiting it for food. The parasite can even take over the host's mind, changing its behavior and transforming it into an apparently different creature with its sole purpose to serve the parasite's needs. These organisms are capable of inducing the host to crave certain foods so that they can continue reproducing, while at the same time starving the host of nutrients and eventually taking over completely. This is an imminent risk we all face. However, it is with the proper diet, that this scenario can be highly prevented.

As an additional note, Carl Zimmer — a scientist writer and author of the earth-shattering book "Parasite Rex: Inside the Bizarre World of Nature's Most Dangerous Creatures" — vividly explains how parasites have the extraordinary ability to rewire the brain and control the minds of their hosts, even changing its genes. This is a book well worth reading.

However, if you're eating a poor diet, are dragged down by stress and anger, and take medications on a regular basis, then you're not giving your army of probiotic bacteria a chance to fight off the enemy. Not surprisingly, yeasts, parasites and pathogenic bacteria love any type of sugars, including high fructose corn syrup, carbohydrates found in all wheat grains and their byproducts, lactose in pasteurized milk and fructose in pasteurized fruit juices, among others. Sound familiar? If these are the foods you're craving the reason is that these are the types of foods harmful organisms thrive upon. By contrast, if your body is balanced there is little chance that these will be the foods you will crave.

Whenever a parasite takes control of your GI tract the foods it thrives on will undoubtedly be the foods you crave. You will then be feeding the enemy, contributing to rapid weight gain and deteriorating health. With each passing day, your friendly microflora becomes weaker and weaker, and the parasites in your body continue building an army of ruthless invaders. This will result in symptoms such as heartburn, bloating, gas, food intolerances, intestinal inflammation and pain, weight gain, junk food and alcohol cravings, achy joints, hair loss, fungus on the nails, ADD, premature aging and so much more.

If you're perplexed about the way you feel or wondering why someone you love always seems out of sorts, this chapter will open your eyes to a brand new world — the sub-world of parasites that can potentially live in the human body and cause mayhem wherever they become established.

This is certainly not a new concept. Conventional wisdom dictates that if you're suffering with gastrointestinal problems and deteriorating health, then you need look no further than your gut. Traditional medicine believes that the digestive tract is where most disease originates, causing a slow descent into illness and with good reason. The mouth is the entrance to the digestive tract and the means for external influences to enter the rest of the body. So don't take what you put into your mouth for granted.

The way many people have always attempted to lose weight has been by starving themselves, eating prefabricated tasteless foods, making every meal a mathematical formula and creating fear based solely on food. They have spent a fortune on powders, miracle pills and empty promises, but at the end of the day all that's left to show for the weight-loss-battle is yet one more failure, disappointment and self-punishment for a perceived lack of will power. With the Yogurt Diet you will learn a new approach. From this point on, you will be able to enjoy fully every meal you eat. You won't ever have to worry about points, calories, fats or carbohydrates. At the same time, you must be very vigilant about the foods you eat and be sure to know who they are really feeding – you and your friendly flora. Otherwise, you may find yourself eating foods that fatten up the enemy, those harmful organisms that have colonized your gut!

Are Gut Bugs Making You Fat?

World-renowned scientists Richard Atkinson and Jeffrey Gordon have been conducting studies on obesity and its causes for decades and, separately, have arrived at the same conclusions. Both disagree with the conventional notion that overeating and lack of exercise are the *only* reasons for being overweight. They even challenge the idea that genes are not to blame for the obesity epidemic sweeping the western world. If genes were to blame, they question how can it be possible that one identical twin can be thin and the other obese when they have the same exact genetic makeup? The answer is the difference in the bacterial composition of the gut flora from one individual to the next, regardless of genes. Some scientists are developing a new, thought-provoking theory that links being overweight to the microorganisms we harbor in the digestive tract. These findings actually rocked my world when I first learned about them because they coincided with my own research and developing theories over the past few years. This theory has proved effective time and again in transforming people's health when they followed the specific Yogurt Diet, which has the ability to put in place a healthy bacterial ecosystem in an individual.

A normal human body is made up of 100 trillion cells. However, only one in 10 of these cells are human, while the rest of the cells in the human body are of microbial origin. That means an astonishing 90 trillion cells in your body come from microbes. Genes are contained within the body's cells, and because we have more microbial cells than human cells, then it so happens that the vast majority of the genes you carry around, in a sense, they are microbial genes and not human genes. A bit shocking, isn't it?

The entire human microflora can be basically categorized under two major groups of organisms — Bacteroides and Firmicutes. Recent studies show that depending on whether a person is thin or overweight, the amount of one group of microbes will dominate the other. If a person is thin, it will have an abundance of microbes from the Bacteroides group, with Firmicutes co-existing in very small numbers. In an overweight or obese person the microbes of the Firmicute family abound in the gut, far outnumbering the Bacteroides group.

One theory is that the bacteria of the obese-causing Firmicute group are involved in energy re-absorption from foods. These types of bacteria have sophisticated mechanisms in place that allow them to survive extreme conditions. The bacterium that results in ulcers (Helicobacter pylori) is part of this group of weight gain-causing bacteria.

This great discovery leads to the thought-provoking concept that the composition of microbial organisms in a host's gut flora determines whether a person is thin or overweight. Scientists accepting this theory believe that in order to lose weight we must deliberately change the balance of the microorganisms we harbor in the gastrointestinal tract, perhaps by matching nutrition to each person's unique makeup of flora in the gut. How is that for a diet, one geared to feed bacteria in the gut?

Doesn't sound very sexy. But these scientists also state that we're years and years away from knowing enough to make this phenomenon happen. Luckily, the answer is right at your fingertips because the Yogurt Diet has beaten them to the punch.

The Yogurt Diet *is* the answer to what scientists are looking for. They have merely posed the salient question: *How about matching nutrition to the microbiota in your gut?* It was a similar question that resulted in the theory of the Yogurt Diet. However, this doesn't mean that each person must follow a very different diet from everyone else, or that in order to be thin you must know from the moment you're born what bugs you have in your GI tract so you can live a healthy life and have a Herculean or Venus body. Every human body is, in essence, the same. We're all made up of bones, flesh, blood, cells and microbes. But each person has unique traits, such as their DNA, and also their gut flora. If we start with the notion that when we are in equilibrium all bodies are physiologically the same, then all it takes for a person who's out of balance is to correct the imbalances — in this case, the harmful microbes that live in your digestive tract and which should not be there — and replace the bad with good probiotic bacteria.

So now you know that all along there has been something else stopping you from losing weight and it had little to do with exercise and starving yourself of the foods your body truly needs. The reality is that once you rebalance the living bugs in your gut, you will rev up your metabolism into the Formula One engine you were really born to have. That is the ultimate goal of the Yogurt Diet.

In the past, no matter what fad diet you've embarked on – no matter what the concept – was not the answer for permanent weight loss and radiant health. The problems we are facing today surrounding our health go well beyond these old tired concepts. Here comes a major one.

Candida Albicans —
A Fat and Disease Promoting Yeast

As you now know, antibiotics, chlorinated water, stress, a sugar-laden diet, high fructose corn syrup, processed foods, lack of sleep and excess alcohol all have an adverse effect on your friendly gut flora, giving way to an increase of harmful organisms in your gut. One such ruthless little conniving organism that proliferates when your protective army of bacteria dies is the yeast Candida albicans, which simply wreaks havoc in your intestinal ecosystem, leading to a downward spiral of health disasters. You will soon get to know these little devils on a first name basis.

Candida albicans is a type of yeast, a microscopic fungus. Yeasts are naturally part of your flora ecosystem; a few are good and others are harmless when kept under control. As a rule, yeasts live in small numbers in moist dark cavities, which your body has in abundance — the mouth, GI tract, vagina, sinuses and other areas. Your good bacteria are always watchful to keep at bay potentially harmful yeasts and suppress their growth. In other words, when the good guys outnumber the bad there's nothing to worry about. It is when you don't take care of your probiotic friends, however, that yeasts can take over, quietly but surely.

In a healthy individual, there is a ratio of 85-15 percent good versus bad organisms. Unfortunately, due to major changes in our modern lifestyles, this healthy balance of bugs is becoming quite rare in developed countries. In fact, it is becoming more common to see an inverted ratio, 85 percent harmful organisms as opposed to just 15 percent good guys. When your body is burdened with so much toxicity, it is hard to keep your healthy gut flora in place. Instead, opportunistic organisms such as Candida see an opening to colonize the walls of your digestive tract and, without your permission, they move in and make your life miserable by promoting excessive weight, inflammation and disease while also creating uncontrollable cravings and prompting you to eat the foods they thrive on — sugar, wheat products, pasteurized milk and fruit juices, wine and beer, among others.

Sadly, the foods Candida and other unfriendly microbes like are the foods widely consumed in our diet today. The ways in which yeasts promote weight gain in the human body is fascinating and really beyond the scope of what many people have been lead to believe. If you are one of those people who have tried every diet plan on the planet, without achieving permanent results, what follows will give you the answers that you've been seeking, as well as a permanent solution to your problem. You will learn how to finally rid yourself of all that undesirable weight for good.

Yeast Fermentation — Extra Calories into Your Body

Lactic acid bacteria (single cell organisms) ferment carbohydrates, proteins and fats as a means to obtaining energy and nutrients and, in exchange, they benefit you, the host, with the healthy byproducts of lactic acid, short chain fatty acids, enzymes and other necessary nutrients. Yeasts, also single cell organisms, have their own fermentation process by which they extract energy from simple sugars in order to feed, reproduce and thrive. Yeast fermentation is the metabolic breakdown of sugars into alcohol and carbon dioxide. They do not, however, ferment proteins, fats and fibers. Their food of choice is plain sugars, the simpler the better.

Yeasts thrive on the foods that most likely make up the bulk of your daily diet, such as sugar, corn and wheat flours, corn syrup, milk, as well as alcohol. If you have an overgrowth of Candida in your digestive tract you're courting potential problems. For example, whenever you consume the aforementioned foods, the yeasts will make sure to extract every possible calorie from the simple sugars you are consuming, turning them into alcohol and gas, and causing the release of many toxic chemicals inside your body. During this fermentation process, yeasts produce extra calories, alcohol and toxins that turn to fat in your body.

Whenever you eat, you consume a certain number of calories, but what determines how many of these calories are really extracted and how much energy is truly produced are the foods you eat and the type of fermentation produced by the organisms colonizing your gut. Therefore, a calorie is not just a calorie. Much depends on who's eating it and whether that person's gut ecosystem is predominantly composed of thin or fat promoting organisms. And it will also determine whether the person has a fast or slow metabolism. Another mystery solved.

In gastronomy, yeasts have several practical uses. The most widely known uses of yeasts, which date back thousands of years, are to make various forms of alcohol. For example, wine is made from yeast fermentation of fruit sugars; to make beer, yeasts use sugars in wheat grains; cane sugar is used in the making of rum; while yeasts metabolize the starchy sugars in potatoes to make vodka. This process is easy and practical because yeasts love simple sugars and they are readily available in all these aforementioned foods. Yeast, of course, is also used in bread making, a process that also involves the fermentation of simple carbohydrates, in this case sugars present in a variety of wheat flours (bleached and whole wheat, spelt, kamut, barley, rye). But one more element is also necessary to make raised breads using yeast, and that is gluten, the protein present in all wheat grains. Without gluten, bread does not rise and won't acquire the doughy and stretchy characteristic that makes bread so delicious. Oat flour, for example, contains no gluten so bread made with it simply won't rise. Wheat and gluten are like two inseparable Siamese twins; they go hand in hand. In bread making, any of these wheat grains can be used because they all offer the benefit of gluten content at various levels.

Yeasts are also used in the process of cheese aging. First, milk is fermented by lactic acid bacteria, the same simple method used in the process of making yogurt. However, it is a variety of yeasts that are introduced in the later aging process, giving different types of aged cheeses distinct aromas and flavors.

What's not surprising, yet very interesting is that the aforementioned foods cause allergic reactions and gastrointestinal problems in susceptible people. If you have noticed that you have allergic reactions to wheat, milk, cheese, wine or corn, the reason is a good old overgrowth of yeast in the GI tract. When harmful yeasts displace good bacteria and spread throughout your gut, the ingestion of aged cheeses, wheat products, beer, wine, vinegar, pickled foods, soy sauce, milk, and others, will create an effect in your body similar to that of bread or beer making. This includes bloating and the release of gas in your belly, which can cause a great deal of pain. In addition, the chemicals released from yeasts fermenting these foods in your gut will trigger an array of health problems — localized fat retention, skin afflictions, depression, fatigue, and a long list of other maladies. In many cases when you go to the doctor he or she can't tell you what's wrong. In other cases, doctors will tell you that all it takes for these problems to subside is to simply stop eating these foods or to take medication, but the bottom line is that they offer no resolution for the long term, and thus no hope to regain your health. However, it is possible that every single one of these ailments can be reversed and eventually disappear completely by embracing the Yogurt Diet.

This eating program has been designed to clear your body of parasites, re-establish your healthy gut flora and rebuild every system in your body by reintroducing nutrients and enzymes. Once you accomplish this goal, everything else will fall into place naturally and your body will be working at its best once again.

The following is a classic example that will clearly show you what happens when an overgrowth of yeasts is present in your belly. It is, essentially, the same process as bread making. There are three main ingredients necessary to make bread — wheat flour, water and yeast. Flours are carbohydrates, which are chains of starch molecules made up of hundreds of sugar molecules. When yeast, water and flour are combined, enzymes activate and initially break down the long chains of carbohydrates into sugars. This is how the fermentation process begins and is the key to making bread. When yeasts eat the sugars present in flour they multiply rapidly, producing carbon dioxide and alcohol as by-products. The carbon dioxide produced is held in by a network of gluten strands, enabling the gases produced by the yeast to spread, which leavens the flour and causes the bread to rise. This is quite similar to what can happen in your belly when you eat wheat if you have an overgrowth of yeast in your gut.

The yeast in your gut feasts on sugars, producing alcohol, carbon dioxide and toxic byproducts. Your belly begins to expand and the gas becomes trapped, just as it does in a loaf of bread. You then get bloated and full of gas, and that's when you begin to feel pain and discomfort in your abdomen. The alcohol and other toxic waste produced during this process enter and circulate into your bloodstream, eventually being stored and trapped in fat cells, and manifesting themselves as fat and cellulite. These toxic substances may make you drowsy or downright tired, moody and achy, some of the same symptoms as when alcohol is consumed. When the process is repeated over and over again, it can cause inflammation in your joints (arthritis), your colon (colitis), abdomen (obesity) and many other parts of your body. The Yogurt Diet will reverse the problems caused by inflammation of various organs and tissues; and that also makes the Yogurt Diet an anti-inflammatory diet.

If Candida or other parasites take over you will gain weight, regardless of how little you eat, because you continue to eat more of the same foods, undoubtedly all types of sugars and products containing gluten and wheat, as well as yeasty foods like beer and wine. The major side effects are due to all the toxins that the yeast Candida emits as it ferments sugars in your GI tract. Over time this can cause recurrent mucosal membrane infections, impairment of the production of certain hormones, loss of hair, fragile nails, impotence, infertility, PMS, depression, a weakened immune system, diabetes, skin disorders, obesity, ADD, inflammation of various tissues and much more. Because this fermentation process is repeated every time you eat the offensive foods, your belly will become larger and larger while the parasitic organisms basically acquire a life of their own inside your body. At this point they will cause you to crave the foods *they* like continuously which, in turn, causes harm to your gut and eventually other organs in your body. The cycle is now in full swing, and no matter how restricted your calories or points are, if you keep eating these yeast fermentable foods and feeding the parasites in your belly all your will power and best intentions will go to waste. Now you are simply encouraging the growth of fat promoting and disease-causing organisms.

Celiac Disease and the Possible Yeast Connection

Celiac disease is presently believed to be caused by intolerance to gluten in *genetically* susceptible individuals, interfering with the assimilation of nutrients from food. This digestive disorder results in damage to the small intestine and mal-absorption. When the villi (the tiny fingerlike hairs that normally allow nutrients to be absorbed into the bloodstream) in the small intestine are damaged and inflamed they become unable to absorb water and nutrients, causing the celiac to be susceptible to a variety of other conditions related to digestion, such as lactose intolerance. So far, the elimination of all gluten in the diet has been the only treatment option for patients with celiac disease and with no hope for a cure any time soon. This is like placing a band-aid on a gun shot wound.

However, the more I learn about this disease and the more I witness my clients completely recuperate from this condition simply by following the Yogurt Diet, I can't help but ask myself what might be the real cause behind this horrible affliction that debilitates millions of children and adults today? And all the answers without question point to an imbalance of the gut flora in the intestines.

I want to remind you that what you are about to read has no backing from the scientific community today, as perhaps this is a question they have yet to consider. However, I feel obligated to inform you of the results many of my clients have achieved following the Yogurt Diet, because this might also be the solution for you if you suffer from gluten intolerance. These results, communicated to me by clients over the years, confirm my long term belief that gluten intolerance may not be so much a function of genes, but the result of environmental factors — most prominently the ingestion of antibiotics, which can kill the entire microflora in the intestines leaving the walls bare and susceptible to damage and inflammation, as well as giving room for the rise of yeasts to colonize and take over.

Again, the following is simply my own theory, but one that you should consider, especially if you or someone you know suffers from this persistent ailment. There is nothing to lose and possibly much to gain. That's because it's entirely possible that the Yogurt Diet is the solution that will allow you to start enjoying delicious pasta and breads once again.

With a growing population all around the Western hemisphere suffering from celiac disease (estimates range from 15 to18 percent), it makes sense that radical questions should be asked in order to find answers for eradicating this ailment. Why, for instance, has celiac disease become so prevalent during the past few decades? What are the real causes for this "gluten intolerance?" Where did this disease come from and why was it almost non-existent some sixty or so years ago? Studies support the theory that some people may be genetically predisposed, but then again, how is that possible if the disease was virtually non existent before the

1950's? Has a "new" gene suddenly emerged that makes *only* Westerners genetically predisposed to celiac disease? This fact alone reveals that celiac is certainly a problem we have somehow created ourselves.

In looking for answers, let's start with a bit of history. Wheat originated from Southwest Asia, later spreading to Ethiopia, India and China, and eventually becoming a staple in the diets of the people of the Mediterranean region as it moved from Spain to Northern Africa, Egypt, Israel, Lebanon, Syria, Turkey, Greece, Italy and France. Humans have been consuming wheat grains around the globe for thousands of years. If our ancestors had experienced any discomforts when eating wheat, I guarantee you that spaghetti Bolognese, pizza margarita and croissants would have been eliminated from the human diet long ago. After all, it is our ancestors who designed diets throughout time on a trial and error basis. Give them some credit. Wheat, in itself, cannot be bad. Rather, it must be something that we're doing that's to blame for the advent and rise of celiac disease.

It stands to reason that if wheat has been eaten safely for thousands of years and celiac disease has only appeared as a major problem in our lives over the past 50 to 60 years, that something is being overlooked. We also know, for instance, that this disorder is virtually non-existent in underdeveloped countries. As we put together all our evidence we have to look for changes that have occurred over the past few decades that can be associated with the rise of this ailment. When I do that, only one answer keeps coming back and staring right at me — a depleted healthy intestinal flora. Perhaps due to the widespread use of antibiotics — literally, the anti-life drug.

Since the commercialization of antibiotics in the 1950's, and as pharmaceutical companies continue to develop more potent varieties designed to kill a larger variety of resistant harmful bacteria, many new diseases seem to be on the rise. Celiac disease is just one of them. The next obvious question is how to connect the dots between antibiotics and gluten intolerance.

As explained earlier, when you take antibiotics the protective army of probiotic bacteria in your gut are exterminated, allowing for the yeast Candida and other parasites to emerge and grow. Now you have a yeast overgrowth in your gut ready to ferment anything that comes its way, and if it's wheat, along with its protein gluten, you now have all the ingredients to make a loaf of bread in your belly. Remember the bread-making example above? It's very possible that the symptoms of a celiac (abdominal pain, bloating, diarrhea, irritability, depression, anemia, stomach upset, muscle cramps, skin disorders, dental and bone disorders) could very possibly be caused by yeast fermentation of wheat in the intestines. The byproducts of this fermentation process are alcohol and carbon dioxide (gas), along with other toxins emitted by pathogenic yeasts. When this type of parasite colonizes any part of the GI tract it can lead to inflammation and the inability to absorb nutrients. This certainly seems like a very plausible theory.

If you have even mild symptoms when you eat wheat, then it's very likely that you have a depletion of gut flora and an overgrowth of yeast in your intestines. The way to reverse this affliction is by eliminating all wheat products and other yeast offending foods (see the list of foods in chapter six) while eating plenty of probiotic yogurt to re-establish your healthy gut flora and health. Once you rebuild your immune system — build up the colonies of healthy gut flora, cleanse your body of harmful yeasts and replace nutrients and digestive enzymes – your tolerance to digest wheat will be restored.

If you suspect that you're suffering from gluten intolerance the first thing to ask yourself is whether you have taken any antibiotics in the past. If the answer is yes, you now know that the Yogurt Diet might very well be the answer that can enable you to reverse these unpleasant conditions — the overgrowth of yeasts in your gut as well as your intolerance to wheat products. *In other words, you can bring your body back to balance with the Yogurt Diet.*

The Low Carb Craze.
It Works, Yet it Doesn't

Many nutrition experts and doctors have been proclaiming for years that we should follow a Mediterranean style diet to be fit and healthy. The basics include eating whole wheat grains with every meal and adding plenty of fruits and vegetables — the wide spectrum of carbohydrates. I would certainly agree that this is basically a very healthy diet. In fact, I have followed it for a good part of my life and can attest to its health benefits, as well as its ability to keep me fit. Then again, I grew up in the Mediterranean, where these foods are served at each and every meal, along with healthy fats and proteins in smaller measures. I have witnessed first hand that people following this traditional diet are quite healthy.

However, as you are beginning to learn, there are many people for whom this wholesome diet might not prove to be so beneficial. In fact, it could even be harmful if their bodies are out of sync. Not only might they experience abdominal and other gastrointestinal discomforts, but they will also gain weight. Why?

Let's take a look at the entire picture. The people of this region who follow a traditional Mediterranean diet have never taken antibiotics in their entire lives, nor have they consumed any quantities of high fructose corn syrup. Sugar is used sparingly with honey as the primary sweetener, and they eat a diet consisting exclusively of whole foods. In essence, this healthy diet works for them because their bodies are in a state of harmony. But look at what happens when you take that harmony out of the equation.

Begin with a childhood diet consisting of sugar laden and processed foods, with a round of antibiotics thrown in here and there. Then as an adult add a few alcoholic drinks most nights, pop in antidepressants, antacid medications, birth control pills and more antibiotics. What you've now done is sentenced your probiotic bacteria to the guillotine and thrown your body completely out of whack. And here's more bad news. Under these conditions the healthy Mediterranean diet will not work for you.

How can this be? Why would something so good for an entire population of millions be so harmful to others? The reason is simple. It's all about maintaining balance of your probiotic intestinal flora. Now you know the harmful effects an overgrowth of yeast can have in your body when you eat certain healthy foods such as whole-wheat grains, wine and the healthy sugars found in milk and fruits. If you're afflicted with an imbalance of gut flora, I regret to announce that the Mediterranean diet is not the appropriate diet for you.

On the other hand, if you eliminate all carbs completely and restrict your diet to only proteins and fats, you will instantly lose weight in your midsection. That's because these types of diets unknowingly, but successfully starve the yeast, which has no more sugars to feed off resulting in their slow extermination. And this is how the "low carb craze" gained its popularity — with claims of "lose your belly fat first." But do these diets really work? Absolutely not! They are a short-lived solution, because the first time you reintroduce any type of sugar, yeasty food or wheat back into your diet, the starving yeasts will ferociously devour these foods, making sure they take over your system once again and the weight will rapidly and surely return with a vengeance.

The Mediterranean diet, of which I'm so fond and highly recommend, will work only – and I emphasize again, ONLY — if and when your gut flora is in place. First, you need that 85-15 ratio of good vs. bad bacteria for equilibrium, and that's exactly what the Yogurt Diet is designed to give you. It's also the reason the people of the Mediterranean stay fit and healthy. Then, once you're done cleansing your system the delicious and healthy Mediterranean diet will certainly work. Bread, pasta, wine, aged and moldy cheeses can all be part of a healthy and balanced diet once you have brought harmony back into your body with the Yogurt Diet.

With the help of yogurt, and other specific foods, this diet is designed to get the bad guys out by starvation, depriving them of the foods they thrive upon. Once you achieve a neutral position within, you'll always be able to keep a slim figure, even if you eat a warm, buttery crispy morning croissant, bread dipped in olive oil for lunch, and a delicious aged cheese with a healthy glass of wine for dinner. This much I promise.

The Yogurt Diet will open your eyes to a brand new approach, one that will give you the answers you've been searching for as well as an understanding of what's happening inside your body. It will also give you the means to put both weight and health problems behind you forever. If you have ever been on a high protein/low carb diet, you will most likely attest that these types of diets work . . . however, only for the short term. Yet in the past few years we have seen the rise of the low carb diet craze, with every modality and style of low carb diet book making their way onto the shelves. Authors, with each personal modification of the "low-carb" diet, have given you their own sensible explanation as to why following their recommendations will allow you to lose weight. Invariably, low carb diets work to initially allow weight loss. The problem arises when you go back to eating certain carbohydrates and the weight returns rapidly and with a vengeance. Then you find yourself struggling to keep the weight off yet one more time, probably with another version of the same diet. This is what has given "carbs" their bad name.

There's a reason why these diets work, but also why they're not the solution to the obesity and disease epidemics that afflict our modern world. None of these diets will ever work for the long run if what you're experiencing is a gut flora imbalance. This is the final word and missing piece to the weight loss puzzle of the twenty-first century. Fortunately, you no longer have to struggle with this unsolved mystery. No diet before has ever addresses the true underlying cause of weight problems triggered by certain carbohydrates. Why do certain carbohydrates promote weight gain while others do not? Why are fruits taken out of the equation in "low-carb" diets, but not vegetables? Both are carbs. The answer is that fruit sugars are fermentable by yeasts, while the long chains of sugars in vegetables are fibers, which are indigestible by those same yeasts but are a true feast for your probiotic flora.

I am far from being another advocate of the low carb craze. I come from a culture where carbohydrates — be it fruits and vegetables, or grain products — dominate every meal. Yet Spaniards are some of the longest living people today, with rare cases of obesity among those who eat the country's traditional cuisine. If you have followed a low carb diet in the past and it worked, great. However, there's a good reason why this book has made it into your hands and why you're reading about the benefits of yogurt. Quite possibly, you're still looking for answers to your weight problems and other ailments that continue to affect your daily life.

That said, there's a logical explanation for the rise of low carb diets in the past decade. The foods that are eliminated in the low carb diets are all types of sugars, including wheat, which are easily fermentable by yeasts, as well as yeasty foods like wine and beer. However, what low carb diets fail to address is the necessity of rebuilding a well-balanced gut flora if you want your weight loss to be permanent and your health optimized. You should now know why these types of diets have been successful in the past, but have never been the answer to the real problem. The cause of weight gain in this case is the overgrowth of yeast. To stop this pattern from becoming a perpetual and frustrating one, pathogenic organisms in your gut need to be replaced by beneficial bacteria. It's really that simple. This is the only way to achieve permanent weight loss.

And so the Damage Begins

When yeasts and other harmful organisms displace the probiotic bacteria in your digestive tract, your immune system becomes slowly compromised. In many instances, instead of rebuilding it with healthy foods and probiotic yogurt, the solution we choose is to pay the doctor a visit for a prescription of antibiotics. This only leads to further weakening the immune system, and it's all downhill from there. The real problem begins when destructive parasites break down the protective mucus layer of the intestines. This allows toxins to penetrate organ tissue before being released and transported into the bloodstream so they can travel throughout the rest of the body causing harm at various locations, depending on the amount of toxins circulating within the system. You may begin to experience an array of discomforts — allergies, hormonal imbalances, an impaired immune system, gas and bloating, heartburn, pain of the joints and inexplicable weight gain et al.

Probiotic bacteria in the digestive tract have sophisticated mechanisms in place that may influence satiety (feeling full), such as the ability to send signals to the brain that let you know you've had enough to eat. But weight-promoting organisms can have the opposite effect. By impairing certain hormones and receptors in your body they prevent you from feeling satisfied. Parasites can be very sneaky and may play a role in making you crave the junk they love, so that they can continue reproducing and growing inside your body. This effectively impairs your "will power" and judgment while promoting even more weight gain. Once these types of pathogenic organisms have taken over they will dictate what you want to eat and how much of it. Your cravings could spiral out of control, with the inevitable result being uncontrollable weight gain. Certain parasites also have the ability to extract and reabsorb energy from the foods you're eating; producing an enormous amount of extra energy in your system that even time invested at the gym cannot burn. And this is just one consequence of a bacterial imbalance in your body.

While you may have thought that it was your lack of will power preventing you from sticking to a sensible eating plan, in reality it could be a bacterial imbalance that is playing a major role in causing you to crave foods that will ultimately hurt your health and weight. In fact, when you are burdened with an overgrowth of parasites, such is the case with yeasts, even so-called "healthy foods"— like whole-wheat grains, wine and fruits — will do more harm than good. And subsequently, your overall health will be compromised as well.

When your system is so far out of balance, you must take absolute responsibility for your own health and actions. Stop taking the easy way out by relying on truckloads of medications and weight loss potions. You must take RESPONSIBILITY. I know this is a big word to swallow, but without taking full responsibility for yourself, you will continue riding on the same circular bus with only one stop: Fiasco. Embrace the Yogurt Diet whole heartedly and seek the guidance of a caring doctor who understands your problem. Don't hesitate to share this book with your health care providers so that everyone is on the same page and he or she can guide you to a healthier lifestyle, while also helping other patients regain their health.

In chapter six you will find a list of the foods that must be avoided when cleansing your body of bad bugs and toxins as well as a list of the marvelous foods you should eat to bring back health and reestablish the good friendly bacteria back into your gut. Learn them and know them well, and I promise you'll be glad you did.

Chapter Five

Probiotics:
A Life Promoting Force and the Burning Engine of Your Metabolism

Have you ever wished you could eat an abundance of delicious foods without worrying about the number of calories you're ingesting? Do you dream of enjoying a magnificent meal for simple pleasure and being able to leave the table without guilt? Would you like to have the fast metabolism that will make it all possible? This chapter will open your eyes to a revolutionary idea that will make it possible for you to never have to worry again about dieting, calories, fats, carbs, points, or the glycemic index.

The days when I struggled with my own weight are now a distant memory. I had moved to the United States as a young student and within nine months put on a horrifying 25 pounds. That event changed my life forever. At the time I didn't think much of it, but eventually the extra weight became increasingly uncomfortable and embarrassing on my small frame. While growing up in Spain I had always been very thin. As a young teenager, I actually felt left out because some of my friends were always on one new diet after another. I would hear them talk about it like it was the fashionable thing to do and I could never join in. At some point I even wished I had been overweight just to reach that level of bonding with the rest of the girls. But when the good old days were over and a real weight problem began, I thought of a very apropos saying. Be careful what you wish for . . .

I, too, wasted many precious years of my life dieting and struggling with my weight determined to never be the girl with the big butt. Years later, while still living in my new found home, the United States, I consciously decided to go back to my Mediterranean roots and start eating all the foods I grew up loving, and which I also enjoyed cooking for my clients as a private chef.

So my journey began. As if by magic my fast metabolism kicked in, showing up with amazing force. As I'd soon learn, it had always been inside of me but I was suppressing it with supposedly "healthy", but never the less poor dietary choices and processed foods. I was fearless with the foods that I would dare to eat without any guilt — croissants, heavy cream and strawberries, butter, lamb and crispy fries fried in olive oil. Needless to say, junk foods of any type were not on the menu, just wholesome, delicious, homemade fare. I began including whole milk yogurt back into my diet, every day, three times a day and just the way I would eat it at home, with seasonal fruits sprinkled with some type of nuts and agave nectar (a new delicious and healthy addition to my diet.) To my surprise I didn't gain a single pound that did not belong on my small-framed body, but even more interesting was the fact that many of my persistent health battles disappeared one by one.

I then began to realize how long I had been punishing my body with near starvation diet techniques only to surrender at the end to overeating unhealthy sugary and processed foods. It was yoyo dieting of the first rank. What was I thinking? Once again, the answers had always been right in front of me. I was simply not asking the right questions and not connecting the dots.

This difficult event in my life led to a strong desire to learn everything there was to know about food and nutrition, as well as how to be fit and healthy. I began studying nutrition at school, but remained unsatisfied with what I was learning in an academic environment. Many of the theories that were being taught contradicted with what I had witnessed as a child and then found through my own experiences with weight loss and health. That's when I began to research and devour every piece of information on traditional world diets and study papers on nutrition by highly regarded scientists from all around the globe. I started reading medical journals and, eventually, my intrigue and love for yogurt lead me to learn about microbiology (the science that studies microbes). That's when a whole new world opened up in front of my eyes. My belly was always full of good food, but my mind was insatiable, always hungry to learn more. After learning a great deal on my own I soon discovered the missing piece in this messy weight loss puzzle afflicting our population today — probiotic bacteria in the gut.

You now know how an imbalance of gut flora can cause chaos in your entire system and allow for the growth of harmful organisms — like killer bacteria, the yeast Candida albicans and countless parasites — that make you crave all the wrong foods and promote weight gain and disease. The next step is to learn how to restore balance back into your body with probiotic bacteria found in yogurt, to speed up your metabolism so you never again have to surrender to depravation diets, and along the way achieve optimum health.

More Reasons to Eat Yogurt

The colonies of healthy bacteria that live inside the GI tract are single cell organisms that perform many functions of immeasurable value connected to the health of the entire body. To refresh your memory, the human body is made up of 100 trillion cells and of those, 90 percent actually come from microbes that live throughout the body. The other mere10 percent are human cells. The reason why I'm reminding you of this is so that you realize how much of you is actually of bacterial origin. Most of the bacterial make-up of a healthy individual is from the bacterial species Lactobacillus, Bifidobacterium and Streptococcus, some of the very same bacteria present in yogurt. No surprise there. The gut flora, however, naturally becomes depleted with age and this is yet another reason it's so important to constantly keep replenishing it with yogurt. This is also a major reason why the people of the Mediterranean and the Balkan regions live virtually disease free deep into old age. They consume live yogurt and kefir, as well as other lactic bacteria fermented products daily.

The following is a list of functions that are dependent upon the gut flora for optimum health and a long and disease free life. They are also major components in achieving ideal weight naturally and without dieting.

1. The Immune System — The gut flora plays an integral role in building a fully developed and competent immune system from birth and then maintaining it throughout your entire life. The part of the immune system located in the digestive tract is the principal line of defense against the different forms of aggression to which the body is subjected every day. Amazingly, 70 percent of your body's total immune system is located right in the digestive tract, where specific friendly bacteria attach themselves to the lining of the intestines, forming a barrier to protect the body against harmful pathogens. Regular consumption of probiotic yogurt helps regulate the level of protective bacteria, reinforcing this barrier and helping to maintain overall health.

When disease-causing agents attack the body the immune system reacts immediately with an inflammatory response, which is a defense mechanism to eliminate pathogens from the body. This reaction, however, must be tightly controlled and the body needs to rapidly return to a balanced state to prevent inflammation from evolving into a chronic inflammatory disease. The microbiota in the intestines provides a strong line of defense, preventing harmful organisms and toxins from passing through the gastrointestinal tract into the bloodstream. Because of this, it is necessary to maintain a high density and tight connection between the bacteria of the gut flora to create a dense wall and keep the bloodstream free of pathogens. The good guys and the bad guys fiercely compete for nutrients, which are present in limited quantities in the intestines. That's why it's important to eat good quality whole foods to keep this army of disease-preventing soldiers well fed and continue replenishing your digestive tract daily with probiotic yogurt.

Some species of the gut microflora are able to inhibit pathogens from sticking to the mucus walls of the intestines by creating an environment that hinders the growth of harmful competitors. There exists a great deal of scientific evidence showing that when yogurt with live active cultures is ingested it has a positive effect on the immune system, increasing antibody and natural killer cell populations. It has also been demonstrated that probiotics are able to produce antibodies precisely directed against specific invaders. Consumption of lactic acid bacteria are known to increase resistance to immune-related diseases, and may lead to remission of colitis, celiac disease, IBD, and other inflammatory diseases in the GI tract; as well as being a preventative measure to many ailments.

With all this exciting groundbreaking evidence it's apparent that a combination of a healthy diet, an active lifestyle and the addition of probiotic yogurt must all become priorities in your life to ensure the body's defense mechanisms are always working properly.

2. Detoxifying Effects of Probiotics — Various species of probiotic bacteria in the colon have detoxifying abilities, and these microbes are involved in the production of specific agents such as detoxifying enzymes, which are used for the breakdown of pollutants and overall purification of the body. This is a system put in place to rid the body of poisonous substances that can adversely affect one's health. The detoxifying enzymes produced by certain colonic species have the ability to inhibit the growth of tumors in different body organs. At the same time they protect all cells from a wide variety of toxins produced from naturally occurring metabolic reactions in the body as well as foreign substances that avertedly make it through.

The gut flora also perform additional detoxifying actions by reducing the concentration of bile acids in the colon, and by diminishing the presence of putrefactive bacteria in body waste, which are responsible for generating disease causing substances. It is of major importance that your colon remains colonized by benign bacteria at all times so that these detoxifying effects can take place every moment of your life. Consume yogurt three times a day to replenish your "microbiota organ" and you will ensure a long and healthy life.

What Are Enzymes

An enzyme is a driving energy that is involved in every metabolic process in the body. All living organisms are a succession of enzymatic reactions. The function of enzymes is to digest all the food you eat and convert it into small enough particles able to pass through the little absorbent hairs of the intestines, the villi, and into the bloodstream. Enzymes in the blood then take the micronutrients of digested food and build it into muscles, nerves, more blood and glands. Minerals, vitamins and hormones interact with various enzymes to fulfill their functions. Enzymes also break down toxic substances so that they can be eliminated from the body safely and effectively.

3. An Optimum Working Digestive System — Digestion is the mechanical and chemical process that breaks down foods. It begins in the mouth and ends in the rectum with excretion. In the mouth, foods are mixed with saliva and enzymes, where the digestion of carbohydrates begins. Then, food is pushed down the esophagus and into the stomach, where proteins, fats and carbohydrates further break down in the presence of gastric juices, more enzymes and the mechanical churning of muscles (known as peristalsis). Once converted into more simple structures, these foods can pass on to the small intestine where the bulk of digestion occurs and the vast majority of nutrients are absorbed into the blood. Some nutrients that cannot be broken down and absorbed in the small intestine — such as indigestible carbohydrates known as dietary fiber, some proteins and lipids — will move on to the colon. Once there, the gut flora ferment and break them down for both their nourishment and yours, and produce essential byproducts from the process of fermentation such as lactic acid and the essential short chain fatty acids which are absolutely needed to maintain optimum health.

There exist somewhere between 300 to 500 different types of organisms in the GI tract; some friendly and others not so amiable. But the fact is that the probiotic bacteria in the gut have an important job to perform. The micro-organisms in your digestive tract are constantly at work, waiting for you to send provisions their way so that they can perform the task at hand. The presence of a desirable digestive flora is essential for proper digestion and optimum health. The different types of bacteria in the digestive tract secrete an incredible variety of enzymes that assist in a long list of metabolic functions. They promote optimum digestion and act as a facilitator to many vitamins, minerals and hormones. The human body lacks many enzymes to digest certain foods, such as fibers, and it is wholly dependent on the production of these enzymes from bacterial fermentation to extract needed nutrients and energy from these foods.

Given what we know so far, it may be safe to say that most digestive problems and food intolerances people experience today have to do with a debilitated gut flora in the GI tract. For example, in the case of milk intolerance the enzyme lactase is needed to digest the sugar lactose present in milk. If the friendly lactic acid bacteria in your digestive system have been replaced by harmful organisms, then most likely the stores of the enzyme lactase have become depleted. If this is the case, then any milk you drink will be indigestible and you will undoubtedly be diagnosed with lactose intolerance. Interestingly enough, even if you suffer from this affliction you will most likely not experience any GI problems related to lactose intolerance when eating the fermented form of milk – yogurt. That's because the probiotic bacteria responsible for turning milk into yogurt — the same kind you would find in your digestive system if properly colonized — have already predigested the lactose for you during the fermentation process, which turns lactose into lactic acid and produces the enzyme lactase.

In addition, the bacteria produce an abundance of enzymes during this metabolic process, which will replenish enzymes back into your digestive system. If you follow the Yogurt Diet this affliction, which was once considered irreversible, will eventually disappear. The wide variety of enzymes produced also improve digestibility of milk proteins and fats. The reason why L. acidophilus is being recognized for its cholesterol lowering activities is because this type of bacteria feeds on complex fats present in milk, breaking down and pre-digesting these lipids into beneficial substances. Probiotic bacteria in yogurt also assist in the increased absorption of calcium, phosphorus and iron into the body, and stimulate the secretion of gastric juices. If you are lactose intolerant, don't panic. It is possible to reverse this disorder by following the very specific Yogurt Diet in order to reacquire the enzyme lactase that your body is missing. Not surprisingly, lactose intolerance is also related to celiac disease (gluten intolerance), irritable bowl syndrome and Crohn's disease. These are all inflammatory diseases of the GI tract that are on the rise in today's industrialized world and which can be easily traced back to a lack of healthy gut flora in the lining of the walls of the digestive tract.

Furthermore, a healthy colon and intestinal regularity are highly dependent on diet as well as the type of microflora colonizing the intestines. Studies show that daily consumption of live active yogurt optimizes digestive function by regulating intestinal transit time. This results in an increase of stool volume and a reduction in stool consistency, which helps in rapid waste evacuation.

In essence, for optimum digestion you need an ideal balance of probiotic bacteria in your system. This will enable you to efficiently digest and absorb all the nutrients you take into your body and to ensure that waste evacuates the colon in a timely manner before you run the danger of it being re-absorbed back into the blood stream, which will lead to toxicity and disease. Without your microbiota organ, many digestive problems can arise that will disrupt your well-being.

4. Weight Control — You will probably be shocked when you learn the full influence of the gut flora in the process of weight management and fast metabolism. Remember, regardless of genetic makeup everybody is born with a revved up metabolism. Fast metabolism is what nature intended, and it works best when the body is balanced. However, when you eat all the wrong foods and follow a sedentary lifestyle you are unknowingly creating a sluggish metabolism, which prompts your body to slow down and age prematurely.

Everybody wishes for a fast metabolism, but most people complain that they don't. Why do some people seem to burn fuel like a Ferrari on a fast track? What do they do differently to have a fast metabolism? Did they simply inherit it? Is it in their chemical make up? And are you aware that fast metabolism is not only necessary for optimum weight, but also for your health and to slow down the aging process? These are all important questions that need answers.

Metabolism is a lot like the engine of a car. Without it, the set of chemical reactions that occur in all living organisms to promote life, grow and reproduce could not take place. During this process one chemical is transformed into another by a sequence of enzymes. Enzymes are essential for the chemical reactions that take place during metabolism, so if there is a lack of enzymes in the body metabolism drastically slows down. Also, during metabolism molecules are broken down into smaller units and release energy. These smaller units are subsequently used as building materials by the body. Because these are complex processes they require a great deal of energy. However, if your body has no useful material from which to rebuild and regenerate due to a poor diet, your metabolism goes into emergency mode and becomes stagnant. That's because the body's major concern at this point is to reduce energy expenditure and slow down the pace of cell reproduction to preserve life. This is the body's way to keep you running with the minimum energy cost. So don't blame your sluggish metabolism on your genes. Given the circumstances, it is doing the best it can for you. Take responsibility and go into action. The reason you have a slow metabolism is due to poor diet and a depleted gut flora.

Metabolism naturally slows down with age and then stops at death, pretty much the same thing that happens with the engine of a car. The natural aging process is intimately related to the pace of metabolism. As metabolism slows down, you need fewer nutrients to keep the body running. So, in a sense, it is metabolism that fuels life. Conversely, if you are in your twenties and have a slow metabolism it means that your entire body is aging prematurely. It's entirely up to you to delay the aging process so you can retain your youth for a longer time by choosing to eat wholesome foods and yogurt, which will keep your gut flora continually replenished and your cells renewing.

When you eat processed and readily digestible foods (I call them "food posers.") that are nutrient deficient, overcooked, pasteurized and dead, sugary, devoid of any enzymes or live bacteria, the only thing remaining to be absorbed are calories. But these are empty calories that add up quickly and offer very little benefit to aid the body in maintaining life. These foods are considered dead because they have no enzymes and no live bacteria, as do all raw and fermented vegetables, fruits and milk. Not surprisingly, dead foods offer no building nutrients to enable cells to regenerate, which translates into that dreaded slow metabolism.

Traditional diets throughout the world, some of which date back thousands of years, confirm that our ancestors fed on mainly two types of foods — **pro**biotics and **pre**biotics. Probiotics, as mentioned repeatedly and with good reason, are foods that have been fermented with lactic acid bacteria and other beneficial organisms — foods like yogurt and kefir. Also sauerkraut, butter, pickles, olives, cured meats, salted fish, miso, kimchi, and many, many others. Fermentation was used as a way of preservation before the advent of refrigerators to permit foods to be stored for longer periods of time. Even to this day, fermentation continues to be a popular way to preserve foods all around the world.

Prebiotics, on the other hand, are foods that have the capability to feed the gut flora because parts of them are indigestible by the human small intestine which lacks the necessary enzymes to break down these nutrients. This not only includes fiber from complex carbohydrates, but also a portion of proteins and healthy fats. These foods are extremely important to your health because as they pass undigested into the colon they serve as nourishment to colonic bacteria which are capable of extracting nutrients that would otherwise be wasted, and subsequently produce enzymes along with other important byproducts essential to maintain life.

Along with their other qualities, prebiotics also improve colon health and immune function. Foods such as oatmeal, whole grain rice, raw and cooked vegetables, fresh fruits, agave, legumes, garlic and olive oil are among the foods that provide nourishment to healthy bacteria in your digestive tract and thus promote their livelihood. On the other hand, simple sugars and processed foods are readily absorbed into the small intestine, leaving no indigestible nutrients to pass on to the colon, thus starving the gut flora of nourishment.

The most exciting news about prebiotic foods might be for those desiring to lose weight simply because they offer a great solution that allows you to eat normal quantities of food while greatly reducing your caloric intake. This may not sound logical, at first, but it's just the way prebiotics work in your body. Humans lack the types of enzymes needed to digest and metabolize a portion of the nutrients present in whole foods. Therefore, when you eat complex foods, a portion of them are not absorbed and metabolized in the small intestine. Instead they pass on to the colon for bacteria to feast on them. This in turn helps reduce the production of glucose, allowing your body to draw stored energy from fat cells. Basically, this is the same concept behind eating a low calorie diet, but much more effective as you will never feel hungry or deprived. The result of not focusing on calories, but rather on eating prebiotic foods and feeding your friendly gut flora has infinitely more health benefits with all the added pleasure.

Look at it this way, when you eat prebiotic foods it's as if someone else is ingesting those extra calories for you, while you're the one enjoying the delicious fare. From now on you can focus on eating not only for your nourishment, but also for the needs of your healthy bacteria. These friendly guys can help you in so many ways that it's now fair to say that they're really the missing piece in the weight loss puzzle.

In chapter six, you will find a long list of foods that you can eat, not only when following the Yogurt Diet, but also for the rest of your life if you want to continue enjoying marvelous food and radiant health. This will translate into saving many, many extra calories and the subsequent weight gain that goes along unhealthy eating.

Hopefully, you now understand that cutting back calories in processed foods is not the solution to the weight battles we face today. Rather it's a matter of eating wholesome foods where many of those calories simply will not count, and the ones that do count will promote

Glucose

This type of sugar results from digested carbohydrates into a chemical that the body can easily convert to energy when needed. Our digestive system uses bile and enzymes to break down the starch and sugar from carbohydrates into glucose, making it readily available to be absorbed through the small intestine into the bloodstream. Glucose serves as the primary energy source for all the body's cells and for brain functioning. This simple sugar is critical in the production of proteins and in fat metabolism. It is also a precursor for vitamin C and other several important substances. The liver and muscles are the short-term reservoir for glucose, while adipose tissue (fat) takes the extra sugar circulating in the bloodstream and acts as the body's long-term energy reservoir converting glucose into fat. If you consistently have more glucose in the bloodstream than you use, the excess will be stored into your body's fat cells translating into weight gain and eventually leading to obesity, diabetes and many other diseases.

health and ideal weight. When you focus on eating prebiotic foods, restocking your digestive system with natural occurring enzymes and replenishing your gut with probiotic bacteria in yogurt, you're a winner in many ways. This is the true path to creating an ultra fast metabolism so you can make weight loss permanent in your life.

5. **Production of Short Chain Fatty Acids (SCFAs)** —You have already heard this substance mentioned throughout as one of the keys to good health. It's time you knew exactly what short chain fatty acids (SCFAs) are and what they can do for you. These substances are extremely important, yet unheard of by most people. SCFAs are a part of the entire chain of events attached to the gut flora, which lead to health and ideal weight, and are exclusively produced in the colon by your gut flora.

The vast majority of SCFAs in the human body derive from the breakdown of indigestible complex carbohydrates, proteins and fats that escape digestion in the small intestine and pass on to the colon to be fermented by the existent healthy microbial populations. The gut flora metabolize unused material to provide energy to all cells in the body. This energy, in the form of SCFAs, is needed to regenerate cells and perform instrumental body functions optimally. Short chain fatty acids are the single most abundant and perhaps most important byproduct of bacterial fermentation, not only because they are a prominent source of energy to every organ in the body (brain, heart, kidneys, muscles, etc.) but also because of the many functions these fatty acids help perform.

The amount and types of SCFAs produced in the colon of a healthy host are determined by diet, microbial factors and intestinal transit time. Conversely, if you lack an abundance of good bacteria in the colon and your diet consists of mostly processed foods that are easily absorbed in the small intestine, no nutrients will remain for the bacteria in the large intestine to ferment with the result being damaged health. Other factors also affect bacterial metabolism and SCFA production in the gut. They include aging, stress, pancreatic and other secretions in the digestive tract, mucus production, disease, drugs and antibiotics.

And just so that you realize the importance of having enough SCFAs produced in the colon, I will tell you that extensive research shows that these substances are essential for general well-being in several different ways. The following is a list of health benefits SCFA provide. This list might be rather technical and quite honestly a bit daunting. However, I want you to try to get over this hurdle and hopefully come away appreciating the mounting scientific evidence that should convince you to take charge and willingly change your eating habits as you embark on the Yogurt Diet. Ready? Here we go.

1. SCFAs produced by the probiotic species Lactobacilli in the gut help lower LDL or "bad" cholesterol. Lactobacilli bacteria is responsible for metabolizing cholesterol into SCFAs, which will then be used by the body as necessary energy.

2. SCFAs produced in the colon also have the ability to reduce blood levels of triglycerides in the blood that are responsible for atherosclerosis.

3. SCFAs play a crucial role in immune protection in two ways:

    a. By lowering the pH in the colon, which makes the environment in this part of the digestive system more acidic, thus preventing the growth of disease-producing organisms.

    b. SCFAs possess powerful antimicrobial activities known to inhibit the growth of undesired pathogens.

4. SCFAs aid in the absorption of nutrients, such as calcium, magnesium, and iron. For example, without a healthy balance of friendly bacteria, no matter how much milk you drink, the calcium just won't be absorbed into your body efficiently if you don't have enough SCFAs being produced in your digestive tract by LAB. Calcium is a mineral that's more soluble in an acidic environment. The production of short chain fatty acids by healthy bacteria in your colon, as well as in yogurt, provides this attractive acidic environment for calcium to be efficiently absorbed into your body.

5. SCFAs encourage the formation of a barrier in the colonic mucosal layer to inhibit inflammatory irritants, which in turn protect the lining from developing colonic polyps (tissue growth in the lining of the colon).

6. SCFAs slow down and inhibit the growth of cancerous cells, protecting the body from colon cancer.

7. SCFAs have the ability to eliminate cancerous cells from the body completely.

8. SCFAs help release insulin from the pancreas, stabilizing blood glucose levels. They also help regulate liver control of glycogen (the form of stored glucose) breakdown.

9. SCFAs are an instrumental part of weight loss because they generate needed energy to burn fat in addition to providing energy to the bacteria in the gut. Without a proper supply of energy the metabolism of cells slows down.

10. SCFAs stimulate leptin expression (the hormone that regulates body weight), contributing to the increase of leptin levels circulating in the body. SCFAs, insulin and leptin are all linked together sending signals and stimulating one another to maintain ideal weight.

There. Now, don't say I didn't warn you. But you made it. And if you're still not sure of the benefits of short chain fatty acids produced by probiotic bacteria in the colon, you might want to read the list again.

Colorectal Cancer

Colorectal cancer is a digestive system disease affecting the large intestine and rectum. Colon cancer in the United States is more prevalent in women than it is in men, and it's the third-leading cause of cancer deaths in women. Digestive disorders such as IBS, ulcerative colitis, polyps and Crohn's disease can all lead to colon cancer. Reestablishing the colonies of probiotic bacteria in the colon and following the Yogurt Diet may be among the most important advice for anyone suffering from any of these diseases; as well as a possible preventative measure or even a potential cure for many bowel inflammatory diseases. The jury may still be out, but please take it to heart. You have nothing to lose and only your health to gain.

Leptin and the Link to Permanent Weight Loss

Leptin is the hormone responsible for regulating body weight. This chemical is produced and released by fat cells in adipose (fat) tissue and is involved in the control of appetite, energy storage and metabolism. Leptin also regulates reproduction and immune response. This weight-regulating hormone travels from fat tissue all the way to the brain, sending messages on nutritional status and fat stores to reduce appetite. Levels of leptin circulating in the body and weight are highly correlated; consequently a lack of adequate leptin levels in the blood result in the hormone's failure to send signals to various systems in the body. We now know that this breakdown in communication is associated with obesity, overeating, infertility and immunological defects. Leptin stimulates the action of the anorexigenic hormone (Neuromedin S) responsible for suppressing food intake and increases levels of another hormone (corticotropin-CRH), also responsible for reducing food intake, in addition to increasing energy expenditure. SCFAs are a high stimulant of leptin production in the body, which also helps with fat oxidation in adipose tissue, resulting in reduced fat mass and body weight. On the other hand, a deficiency of leptin is associated with fat accumulation and weight gain. Fasting and starvation *also* severely decrease blood leptin levels. What this means exactly is that whether you're overeating junk or starving yourself on a crash diet the outcome is a decreased concentration of leptin in the body. Now you know that both scenarios lead to insufficient leptin and poor satiety signaling to the brain. In either case, this translates into overeating. This connection may explain yet one more reason for the high failure rate of dieting, as low leptin circulating in the blood is likely to be a potent stimulus for weight gain.

I hope that having read everything up to here, you now understand fully just how important it is to treat the body as a whole and not in bits and pieces.

The connection between SCFAs in the colon being responsible for the stimulation of leptin production is yet one more reason to believe in the great importance of the gut flora as the means to achieve ideal weight naturally and effortlessly. This is simply one more little piece in the entire chain of events that take place in your body every breathing moment. Therefore, when looking into the various systems and their functions the focus should be on achieving balance by recognizing the body as a whole — not as separate elements — where every piece works together to produce a cascade of effects. It's all about harmony. When once piece falls out everything else can easily come apart as well. The body is a complex entity and each piece of this perfectly designed machine must fit together flawlessly.

It certainly makes sense that you must eat a healthy diet to nourish your body and also replenish your gut flora daily with probiotic yogurt if you want to find balance and achieve ideal weight, while enjoying delicious foods at the same time. The majority of diets simply don't address this balancing act. Diets are like a circus juggler balancing a stack of dishes over his head while riding on a one-wheel bicycle. One wrong move and everything crashes into a million shattering pieces.

Remember the story I told you earlier about Rosa and her plan to gain weight for her wedding day by depriving herself of the luxurious Spanish siesta? As silly as it may have sounded, there's actually a scientific explanation. It is the leptin hormone which is believed to be the connection between lack of sleep and obesity. The levels of this weight-regulating hormone increase about 30 percent while you're in a deep sleep. If you have problems catching your zzzz's, leptin volumes decrease, resulting in lower leptin levels in the body which, in turn, stimulate appetite and promote the inevitable weight gain.

If what you're looking for is permanent weight loss and radiant health, it makes sense to first bring the body into harmony with good amounts of healthy home cooked foods and probiotic yogurt. Then, in time, everything else will fall into place, naturally and effortlessly. This provides additional evidence that losing weight is not as simple as just counting points, calories, fats and carbs. You have to fully understand that the body is a string of reactions and events where every function is dependent on another and all must work together for ultimate success. It's all about balance. I can't say it enough!

Get Your Probiotics from Dairy Yogurt

A good quality yogurt with live active bacteria is the quintessential probiotic, a true functional food consumed by our ancestors for thousands of years. The average amount of probiotic bacteria in yogurt is about 100 million per gram. A serving of yogurt is typically 5 ounces, and there are approximately 142 grams in this size serving. That means that when you eat one single serving of yogurt you're consuming a whopping 14 billion bacterial cells. Imagine the great health benefits when you consume yogurt three times a day, as the Yogurt Diet recommends.

Sometimes, along with the yogurt symbiosis (Lactobacillus bulgaricus and Streptococcus thermophilus), other bacteria are also added, such as Lactobacillus Casei, L. acidophilus L. rhamnosus, L. Burgaricus, L. Salivarious, , L. rhamnosus and Bifidobacteria. The Bifidobacteria, which are not strictly speaking LAB, such as Bifidobacterium breve, or B. bifidum, are also frequently found in many fermented milk products. Okay, time to get over how difficult the names may be to pronounce. What really matters is that their benefits are endless.

The viability of a probiotic to produce its full health potential is dependent on several factors and simply ingesting it is not good enough. Many things must come into place. The bacterial cells need to remain active and alive throughout the digestive tract to promote its health-giving qualities to the consumer. Careful studies demonstrate that after consuming a good quality yogurt, significant growth of health-promoting bacteria in the gastrointestinal tract occurs. However, this is not always the case with other inexpensive probiotic products packed in concentrated forms of dried bacteria in capsules or tablets commonly sold at drug stores. It doesn't necessarily mean that there aren't any good neutraceutical probiotics on the market — there certainly are — but they can come at a hefty price. Consuming yogurt for its proven probiotic benefits is not only much more economical, but also delicious and it leaves open the option to add other healthy ingredients that compliment the nutritional value of yogurt. And that's not even mentioning all the other health benefits you reap from the nutrients present in milk.

It is important to keep in mind the viability of the live bacteria or your best efforts as well as your money will go to waste. There are a number of factors that are necessary for probiotics to effectively deliver their therapeutic benefits to the body. For openers, if you buy yogurt, a precise packaging method must be followed for the bacteria to survive shelf life. Then the bacteria must be able to survive the acids in the stomach as well as other physiologies occurring in the digestive tract. Bacteria need very rigorous growth conditions to reproduce and form clusters of cells binding together to ensure that they will survive the aggressions of digestion and will be able to colonize the GI tract.

The survival of the live bacteria therefore depends on the following conditions:

1. **The medium** in which it is fermented. Milk is the preferred medium for lactic bacteria.

2. **The vector** is the number of cells per gram and the velocity in which they travel the digestive tract. This, too, is very important.

3. **Ability to survive** gastric acids, bile salts and pancreatic secretions.

Studies demonstrate that dairy products act as a preventative barrier between various types of probiotic bacteria and stomach acids. For this reason it makes sense to consume your daily doses of probiotics from yogurt or other milk fermented products.

Peristalsis (the repetitive contraction of muscles in the digestive tract which moves food forward) is also important because it allows for food and bacteria to move rapidly throughout the first part of digestion, until it reaches the colon, where transit time is necessarily slower. Therefore, the vector plays a vital role in the survival of ingested probiotic bacteria.

Whey and Lactoferrin

If you are not convinced yet, let me give yet two more major reasons to acquire probiotics from yogurt – whey and lactoferrin (LF), the two major proteins in milk. Whey is quite a more complex protein as it is made up of many smaller proteins. One of these is the superstar LF, found only in mammals' milk. Human breast milk is most abundant in LF, followed next by cow's milk. LF is found throughout the human body in small traces and is also present in secretions that bathe mucus membranes such as saliva, tears, nasal and bronchial secretions, pancreatic fluids and semen. LF is a multitasking protein with well-recognized antiviral, bactericide, fungicide, anti-parasite, anti-inflammatory, antioxidant, and anticancer activities; as well as having immune-enhancing effects. The immune defense promoting properties of LF might be due to its ability to absorb iron, a most essential mineral for all living organisms, including dangerous microbes. Many pathogenic bacteria need a supply of free iron to multiply, but lactoferrin's ability to bind iron and put it out of circulation may account for some of its antimicrobial functions and immune response capabilities. LF inhibits viruses by binding to viral receptor sites, therefore preventing the virus from infecting healthy cells. In lab studies, LF has been used as a natural antibiotic to treat bacterial infections that cause ulcers and urinary tract infections (UTI). Also, when LF was fed to healthy humans, it showed an extraordinary increase in friendly gut flora and a decrease of some species of harmful bacteria, virus and fungi. It may be interesting to note that the yeast Candida albicans was among the microbes studied. However not every pathogenic microbe can be inhibited by LF.

LF, specifically from fermented yogurt, also has antioxidant capabilities to diminish oxidative stress to tissues from the removal of free iron (a major contributor in the generation of free radicals and a cause of cancer) from circulating in the system. This action prevents premature aging and deterioration of organ tissue and cells. All this continues adding to the list of reasons the people of the Mediterranean are among the longest living and healthiest people in the world.

The Milk Controversy — Get The Facts Straight

Does milk contribute to obesity? This is a question which has led to a great deal of debate lately. There are even instances now where concerned parents and/or health authorities are strongly opposing to milk in children's diets. They've come to believe that milk is not only unhealthy but a major contributor to childhood obesity, allergies and other illnesses proliferating among the younger generation.

But look at it this way. Humans have consumed milk and its derivatives since the beginning of time and it has promoted both life and health to those who were fortunate enough to have it. If milk were bad for our health, our ancestors would have stopped consuming it long ago. That's not the case, however. The bottom line is that milk is a complete and healthy food rich in vitamins, minerals, carbohydrates, proteins and fat. What we need to understand is that the problem is not with mammal's milk. Problems arise when there are microbial imbalances within our bodies, or the cows have been treated with antibiotics and growth hormones. That's when milk can cause trouble, not just promoting allergies, but also weight gain and disease.

For years now we have also been told that fat in milk leads to unwanted weight gain, the very reason today, milk is offered in low-fat and fat-free alternatives. Drinking milk this way is a big mistake. The fat in milk is very necessary for your overall health. Think about it. Would nature have presented this perfect food to us in its whole form if a healthier alternative was low or no fat versions? For starters, the very important vitamins A and D are fat-soluble vitamins in milk and are found in the fat. When the fat is removed these vitamins need to be added from synthetic sources. That's just not the same thing. Both of these vitamins, along with calcium and protein, need to be in the presence of fat in order to be absorbed and assimilated by the body. When you exclude the fat, you're robbing your body of very important nutrients. And remember, your gut flora converts these lipids into much needed SCFAs. So you really have nothing to worry about. After all, the fat content in milk is a mere 3 percent. Did you even know that? What's 3 percent fat in the overall scheme of things? Not very much.

However, there are some circumstances in which milk can lead to weight gain, but it's not because of the fat. Rather, it's the abundance of milk sugars, namely lactose. That is the culprit. At the same time, however, lactose is also an important component of milk and a necessary part of the wholeness of this nutritious food.

For those individuals who have an overabundance of fat promoting pathogenic organisms in their guts, lactose is a perfect food for feeding the enemy. It promotes the continued growth of parasites, thus encouraging weight gain, especially in your midsection (your gut). If you believe the widely spread notion that whole milk is bad and remove the fat, the result is a boost of sugar that will continue feeding pathogenic organisms.

The solution to resolving this apparent problem is to consume whole milk in the form of yogurt. The probiotic bacteria in yogurt offer the benefit of having predigested the sugars and fats for you, while it also comes packed with plenty of enzymes to restore a possible deficit in your digestive system. If you wish to enjoy milk again without running the risk of weight gain and intolerance, follow the Yogurt Diet to reestablish harmony in your body. When you achieve this stupendous balance of microbiota and enzymes, you will be able to drink whole milk without putting on weight or feeling any discomfort. Are you beginning to get the picture? This is one of the many examples showing why enzymes and probiotic bacteria present in yogurt and in your digestive tract are of major importance to your health and weight.

Yogurt — Nature's Perfect Food

If you had any doubt about consuming yogurt made from mammal's milk, this chapter should have answered all the important questions while erasing any semblance of doubt from your mind. Milk is one of the healthiest foods the universe has to offer, especially when it comes from animals that have been treated fairly and fed an appropriate diet free of growth hormones and antibiotics. There's good reason why in India the cow is considered a sacred animal. The best nutrient a cow has to offer is milk which, when raw, just as mother's milk, contains much of life's promoting probiotic bacteria and nutrients. Once milk is pasteurized and the fat removed it loses many of its health benefits, including naturally occurring healthy bacteria, vitamin A and D; but turning whole milk into yogurt returns many of those benefits, once again making milk the perfect food nature intended it to be.

Yogurt and Gingivitis

Do you think you can handle one more reason to eat yogurt? How about a beautiful and healthy smile? A study, led by Dr. Yoshihiro Shimazaki and his colleagues in Japan, has proven that eating yogurt regularly makes a significant difference in periodontal health. Gum disease is a bacterial infection that ultimately leads to tooth loss if not properly managed. Dr. Shimazaki originally set out to find a possible connection between the use of dairy products and a lesser incidence of periodontal disease. He and his team of researchers were surprised to learn that among all dairy products it was actually yogurt that significantly slowed down or stopped this oral disease by the introduction of probiotic lactic acid bacteria (namely Lactobacillus) into the system. It makes perfect sense that if the beneficial bacteria present in yogurt can displace pathogenic bacteria everywhere else in the digestive tract, why not also in your mouth? The research also confirmed that pasteurized milk alone does not have this same effect, as it is the live and active bacteria that promote such great results in ensuring a stunning smile. The scientists also found an apparent lower incident of periodontal disease among people who eat yogurt daily.

Chapter Six

Detoxify Your Body
to Achieve Total Balance

Over time, I have worked with people from all walks of life — no matter their race, sex, age or size — who have suffered for years from many of the long list of previously mentioned ailments. The Yogurt Diet has proven to be the remedy needed to reverse many of these ailments, in most cases causing them to disappear entirely and allowing the previously afflicted people to live completely normal and healthy lives. Eating probiotic yogurt regularly not only allows people to put these health problems behind them, but also prevents new ones from appearing. The Yogurt Diet is not only an answer to obesity and many other ailments. It is also the key to preventing numerous diseases.

The secret to ideal weight and radiant health is in the body's harmony. Ancient medicine adhered to this principle, but it can only be achieved when the body has the right balance of bacterial flora, adequate amounts of vitamins and minerals, plenty of enzymes, energy, amino acids, and other of life's building blocks. When the body's harmony is damaged it must be brought back into balance by eating wholesome and live foods, not by counting calories, fats and carbs, or by eating prefabricated foods and ingesting drugs. And always think yogurt.

Detoxify and Replenish
the Body for Super Results

There's a very sound explanation for why we become overweight and develop disease. Simply put, our body becomes toxic, filled with pathogenic substances and micro-organisms as the result of years of abusive behavior due to stress, lack of sleep, processed foods, excessive alcohol, sugar and chemical laden sodas and sports drinks, taking antibiotics and other drugs, and ingesting a large number of toxic chemicals present in poor quality foods.

An overweight body is simply the reflection of what it looks like inside — inflamed, unbalanced, toxic, chaotic, malnourished and abused. Unfortunately, when we gain weight we often put our entire focus and effort in the wrong place — on our outward appearance. Instead of seeking the real reasons for this unwanted weight gain and overall decline in health, most people simply try to hide behind strenuous diets and medications that ultimately make things worse. The Yogurt Diet is different because it focuses on the problem at hand. Have you ever asked yourself questions like, "Why am I overweight? Why don't I feel my best? Why don't I have energy? Why am I aging prematurely?" You must have the answers if you are to succeed in turning your health and life around.

What I've learned from many years of personal experience, coaching clients and reading through scientific research is that the reason for these problems is almost always the same. When your body begins to accumulate sudden excess weight and your health deteriorates for no apparent reason it is invariably the result of two things — excess toxins accumulating in your body and your gut flora being totally out of balance, often with the good bacteria on the brink of extinction. This is the tipping point that begins creating a serious cascade of effects in all systems of your body and the time when various ailments begin to arise. The Yogurt Diet can be viewed as the missing piece, offering answers to the questions scientists, researchers, doctors, nutritionists and dietitians, as well as so many overweight individuals have been seeking for a lifetime.

That's why the immediate goal of the Yogurt Diet is to purify and replenish the body in order to bring it back into absolute harmony, and this is achieved by eating very specific foods including, of course, probiotic yogurt.

Raw foods and vegetables that have been fermented with live probiotic bacteria have one thing in common. They preserve the healthy organisms that grow naturally on them, which in turn replenish the gut flora, as well as enzymes, vitamins, minerals and antioxidants. This is why it is so important to eat plenty of uncooked fresh vegetables and non-pasteurized fruits or juices, especially during the process of cleansing and detoxifying the body. Remember, enzymes and bacteria break down toxic substances so that the body can eliminate them without damaging the organs and systems. When your body begins the detoxification process, all systems work in unison to eliminate waste through the skin, sinuses, kidneys, lungs and bowels. Your immune system and enzymes become extremely busy breaking down accumulated toxins so that the body can safely and efficiently rid itself of them.

Major Health Consequences From Lack of Bacteria and Enzymes

When you eat mostly processed, overcooked, pasteurized and canned foods the digestive system is constantly taxed and forced to produce an incredible amount of enzymes on its own. This causes the body to draw from its reserves of enzymes stored in organs and tissues, the result being a metabolic deficit. And when the body lacks a healthy bacterial balance and the proper enzymes, it cannot digest food efficiently or absorb nutrients as it should, with the result leading to

A Word of Warning

One must also understand that, as the body begins to mobilize toxins out of your system, it is normal to develop some symptoms such as skin rashes, over-production of mucus, tearing, headaches, constipation, soft stools and urinary tract infections, among others. This is your body's innate natural response, just as your body develops a fever when challenged by a bacterial or viral infection.

The symptoms may resemble those of the flu, but don't give up too soon because you don't feel well. A toxic body is like a sewer that has been backed up for years. When you finally unclog a sewer everything comes rushing out at once, often making a big mess that neither looks nor smells pretty. This is essentially the same thing that happens with a toxic body as it's becoming "un-clogged" of toxins. You have to trust your body and know that the sick feeling is a good sign that all your systems are taking care of business, and that your body is going through a major cleansing. Be resilient, because I guarantee you that it will get better.

a downward spiral of health problems. Unassimilated proteins, yeast cells, carbohydrates and fats are now reabsorbed into the bloodstream causing all sorts of allergies, skin problems and inflammatory diseases in many parts of the body.

In controlled studies, when patients having food allergies were given raw foods and yogurt containing natural enzymes, blood level enzymes returned to normal and their symptoms related to the allergies subsided. Those who regularly eat wholesome foods and include plenty of raw fruits, vegetables and yogurt in their diet can attest to having conquered many illnesses from food allergies, to coronary heart disease, diabetes as well as a variety of cancers. This miraculous outcome is due to the abundance of bacteria and enzymes present in raw and naturally fermented foods containing beneficial live active bacteria.

For thousands of years civilizations around the world, including Greeks, Romans and Egyptians, tribes in Africa and Asia, and in the ancient Middle East have all consumed fermented foods, such as yogurt and kefir, kimchi, salted fish, olives, sauerkraut, miso, cured meats, cocoa and many more. We have our ancestors to thank for providing us with these wonderful healthy foods. Fermentation with probiotic bacteria may be an ancient practice, but what is new are the major discoveries in the past 100 years that point to these types of foods — specifically fermented milk products — as the phenomenon behind the long and healthy lives of people around the world, especially those living at a time when medications were virtually non-existent. Sadly, modern diets have eliminated these super foods, which are rich in probiotic organisms and abundant in enzymes, antioxidants, vitamins and minerals, while replacing them with processed and dead "food posers."

Why are probiotic fermented foods called super foods? There are two major changes which take place in fermented foods that elevate them to this exalted position.

1. The enzyme content in fermented foods can increase up to ten times from their raw counterparts. The plentiful enzymes ensure that your digestive system gets restocked, and your digestion and metabolism work at optimum capacity, resulting in great health and ideal weight.

2. Foods fermented with probiotic organisms are broken down into simpler nutrients, making them more easily digestible. During the metabolic process of fermentation, bacteria breakdown whole foods into amino acids, and more digestible sugars and fatty acids, all of which relieve much of the digestive burden from the body.

Getting Started on the Yogurt Diet

Most people who are overweight with unbalanced bodies eat a large amount of packaged and highly processed dead foods devoid of minerals, vitamins, antioxidants, enzymes and live bacteria. They also consume an assortment of drugs regularly in order to feel better and then go on with their normal lives. All of this affects the gut flora balance and cellular metabolism in a negative way. Because people have lived this way for so long it's completely understandable that the hardest thing to do when trying to implement a new food health plan is to change these old habits. This, then, will be the biggest challenge you'll face when embracing the Yogurt Diet. But just like that fabulous new pair of designer shoes that you have to wear a few times before they feel totally comfortable, you'll soon realize that this new eating style fits you perfectly and naturally.

The Yogurt Diet will allow you to abandon the eating patterns that have controlled your life for so long. The only requirement you'll encounter with the Yogurt Diet is that you must enjoy wholesome and fresh foods from the long list of ingredients included in this chapter, and that you add three servings of probiotic yogurt a day. Think about it. That really isn't a very difficult thing to do.

At the same time, it's not always easy to change eating habits popularly embraced for so many years (such as the notion of counting calories and eating packaged low fat processed foods) and begin adhering to the bolder concept that calories don't matter, and that fat is good for you as long as the foods you're eating come from wholesome and nutritious sources. Please don't fear this controversial idea, because what the Yogurt Diet is proposing is far from a fad diet that will disappear tomorrow. The dietary recommendations presented in the Yogurt Diet are based on traditional diets from around the world that have a long record of proven results. This diet has brought health and longevity to the people who have followed it for centuries. What the Yogurt Diet proposes is a simple concept: cleanse your body and adopt a traditional way of eating. Its sole objective is to take your body on a wonderful journey back to health and ideal weight.

In fact, the Yogurt Diet will allow you to achieve so many fabulous results that you may want to use it many times over throughout your long and healthy life. Initially, when you begin following the Yogurt Diet, your immediate goal might be to lose weight and regain your health. But I guarantee you that once you've achieved your targeted weight many of the lessons learned along the way will remain with you forever. From this point on, whenever you feel your body is veering towards imbalance you'll know exactly what to do.

I have been following this rebalancing diet for years. With the arrival of spring each year, I practice a total body spring-cleaning for three weeks, coinciding with all the fabulous and colorful seasonal fruits and vegetables that appear in the local farmer's markets. I cannot begin to tell you what a difference this yearly ritual makes in my life. My internal engine undergoes a full tune-up just in time to be re-energized so I can enjoy fully the many outdoor activities I love so much. The amount of energy I have is UN-BE-LIE-VA-BLE! And this simple yearly routine also allows me the freedom to indulge in all my favorite foods, like the entire spectrum of cheeses, hot milk chocolate, wine, croissants and breads the rest of the year without gaining a single pound. And, as a bonus, it also gives my immune system that extra boost to ensure I rarely, if ever, get sick.

How Long You Will Need to Stay On The Yogurt Diet

How long you'll need to stay on the Yogurt Diet can be determined by the degree of imbalance present in your body at the time you begin, and then how long it takes for your body to completely detoxify and once again find harmony. This can be accomplished in a matter of weeks, but it can also take several months depending on the state of your body. Don't become discouraged if you need to stay on the Yogurt Diet a bit longer than your best friend, co-worker or spouse. Remember, you are reversing and removing toxins that have accumulated over many, many years. Keep focused, find encouragement from those who love and care about you, and know that at the end you will feel better than you have felt in recent years. By learning to embrace a new lifestyle, you will be undertaking a great accomplishment, one that will allow you to take care of your health without medications and enjoy life to the fullest.

Following the Yogurt Diet will help you shed pounds even as you eat substantial portions of wholesome foods. This is the body's positive response to eating a natural diet, with yogurt leading the way as a conduit to eliminating toxins. Your colon will especially experience a major transformation, as this is the main evacuation organ in the body. Pathogenic substances and organisms harbored in your body for years will be excreted through the colon, helping it to start working optimally as you come closer to a balanced body.

Also of crucial importance is the fact that with the Yogurt Diet you will be starving harmful yeasts, bacteria and parasites as a first step toward eliminating them. This will have a double impact on your weight. One, these pathogens will no longer be growing in your belly, accumulating fat and adding extra calories in your system; and two, as the parasites exit your body you will no longer crave the mostly sugary junk "food posers" you always craved before and which, if you think about it, have constantly sabotaged your best intentions in the past.

Once you complete the initial phase of rapid waste evacuation from your system, you will begin to feel much better and have more energy than you've had in years, and you will continue losing weight. At this point you will be well on your way to building a fast metabolism as you replenish the healthy gut flora, enzymes, minerals, vitamins, antioxidants and everything else your body needs.

I recommend that you do not put a number on the pounds you would like to lose, nor even a time frame because, in reality, these things are irrelevant. Nature takes care of itself and your body knows much better than you do where it should ultimately be and how long it will take to get there. Some people who have been overweight for many years are satisfied losing 60 pounds. For them, this is already a blessing. But they can always be pleasantly surprised to drop an extra 10 pounds they didn't dream would be possible. Others have unrealistic expectations and decide they want to be as thin as some of the so-called supermodels they see on television. My advice is not to fight with what nature gave you. Instead, just embrace it and make the most from it. Look at it this way. **Good health is the new thin!** Once you change the relationship you have with your own body, you will fall totally in love with it!

I also recommend that those beginning the Yogurt Diet take it one day at a time, just ease into it. Don't become discouraged if you find you aren't following it to perfection from day one. Besides its obvious health benefits, this diet is also about making lifestyle changes, and no permanent change can ever be made in a day or two, or even in a week. It takes practice and perseverance because you are in the process of transforming not only learned behaviors, but also your entire relationship with food. By maintaining your commitment to change you will eventually become more of a health conscious person and continue your new lifestyle willingly. Remember, practice makes perfect.

Look at it this way. You cannot say that you're a tennis player unless you play, and play regularly. You can talk about playing tennis all you want, but until you get on the court with your racket and hit some balls with a partner, you aren't a player. It's all about the doing. Changing your lifestyle when it comes to food takes some planning and a resolve to stick with it. Becoming healthy and fit is no different from becoming good at a sport, or even playing a musical instrument. You need to practice daily, have the right equipment at your disposal and hopefully receive encouragement from those around you. That's the only way to do it. Just be committed and continue, every day, every week, every month and every year. You are forging a new lifestyle, one that will be well worth the effort, and one you'll practice for the rest of your life.

Don't embark on the Yogurt Diet because you have a wedding or your ten-year class reunion in two weeks. The Yogurt Diet simply is not meant to be a quick fix. So if you make the decision to join in this wonderful journey, then jump on it wholeheartedly, because it will be totally worth it. You owe it to yourself, and there simply is no better reason than that.

Now let's get started. First you need the tools, in this case a stove, pots and pans, kitchen utensils, recipes and wholesome ingredients. Then you need to learn and practice technique until cooking homemade meals becomes part of who you are. At the beginning, cook a couple of days a week and before long you'll find you're not only doing it every night, but looking forward to it as well. At some point you won't even recognize your old self, the person who used to buy all kinds of packaged foods and keep a variety of sugary and chemical-laden snacks in the pantry, as well as a quart of ice cream in the freezer.

The recipes in this book are so easy and tasty that you don't have to worry about needing the skills of a master chef. You simply have to begin honing your skills no matter what level you're at, and before you know it you'll be catering your cousin's wedding reception. Okay, maybe not quite that large a gathering, but you certainly will be capable of impressing your guests at a dinner party.

What you can look forward to is achieving harmony within every system in your body and feeling absolutely amazing, no matter your age. When you achieve this goal you'll feel completely alive . . . and better than you have in years. That's a guarantee. By that time your body will finally be ready to begin adding back foods into your diet one at a time. So by all means enjoy a glass of wine with cheese and a plate of pasta. Or you might even choose to continue eating this way for the rest of your life and only occasionally eat some of the foods on the *Foods to Avoid* list. While following the Yogurt Diet your body will go through such a miraculous transformation that, even after a few weeks, you will no longer crave many of the foods you've been addicted to for years. Don't expect to crave fast foods or low quality chocolate and machine manufactured pastries. You'll soon find that these foods actually become unbearable to your palate and unimaginable to eat, because they are made with the lowest quality ingredients available. Instead, you will demand your breaded chicken tenders to be fried in extra virgin olive oil, drink only the purest high-grade cocoa, and eat pastries from a local baker made with the best ingredients and loving hands. These foods are so delectable and rich in flavor that a simple bite will send every one of your taste buds into ecstasy. Once your body is completely balanced you will look forward to delicious and wholesome indulgences, rather than the super processed machine made junk you once enjoyed before the Yogurt Diet era began.

A Word About Cheating

There are many terrible diets on the market that call for what I consider classic methods of starvation, as well as other downright unhealthy recommendations. But one of the most laughable behaviors is the notion that someone following a diet "cheats." I find it almost comical when people say, "I'm on a diet, but today I'm going to cheat." What does that really mean? Who are you cheating exactly? The answer to that is easy. You're only cheating yourself. And what are you exactly cheating yourself with? Are you not eating something that's good for you, or are you sneaking something you know is bad for you? Or maybe both? Let's analyze this behavior.

One dictionary meaning of cheating is: *To deceive (betray) or mislead (mis-inform) somebody, especially to gain an unfair advantage.* If this is true, then who is that somebody you're betraying and misinforming? It must be you. So when you cheat, you are deceiving and misleading no one but yourself. Why would you want to do that? When you go on a diet it's usually because you want to lose weight in order to feel better about yourself. Thus when you cheat, stray from the strict guidelines of the diet, you're betraying your word and losing sight of the goals you set out to achieve. That's when you must stop short and ask yourself why you feel compelled to do this. The truth is simply that people cheat in life because they are dissatisfied with their present circumstances or want to gain an advantage at any cost, even if it means being dishonest. Also, when you're following a diet in which you always feel deprived and hungry – which is the case with most of them – there's no question that you will feel compelled to cheat. People are driven by their needs and desires, and when very important needs such as food and hunger are not fulfilled, WE CHEAT!

Diets based upon eating very few calories and processed foods lacking nutrients will always lead to cheating because the dieter is dissatisfied with foods that taste like cardboard. When body and soul are being starved of vitamins, minerals and other important nutrients it's natural to be unhappy and begin looking for other ways to find satisfaction. If a diet doesn't promote self-love and compassion, radiant health and balance then you also cheat and once again betray yourself.

None of these diets can possibly lead to anything positive because there is no long-term satisfaction or life-changing event that you can feel or even sense. The Yogurt Diet is, in itself, a life event. In a way, it's like the day you get married. You make a choice and commitment, and you stick with it. So there's no cheating in the Yogurt Diet. The concept itself does not exist, because the Yogurt Diet is about nurturing and satisfying your needs. It's about loving yourself, no matter what. It's also about embracing the fact that what's happened to you is nobody's fault, but it's certainly within your reach to make the changes that will bring you back to radiant health. The Yogurt Diet is about embracing wholesome foods and putting all your passion into your new lifestyle, even when things are not going well. As with any relationship you value in life, you stay with it because there's a special commitment and bond that you have forged. Cheating is simply dishonest. If for some reason you have to break your routine, it's okay; just return to it right away. But don't think of it as cheating. There's no need to be so hard on yourself when you're on the Yogurt Diet.

Create a Healthy Relationship with Food

The relationship you have with food is perhaps the most important element when you begin looking to change your eating habits. I can't emphasize enough how extremely critical this is. Without transforming your relationship with food you will likely continue to repeat old patterns, and your weight loss will never be permanent. I can attest to this personally. During my formative years everything I learned about food was positive. Food was love, fun, celebration and health. Some of my fondest memories almost always revolved around food — at family gatherings on Sundays cooking the national Spanish dish, paella; barbequing lobster and rabbit with dad; hot chocolate and churros in early morning with friends; birthday parties, weddings, Christmas, learning to cook and spending endless hours in the cozy kitchen with mom; seeing grandma in her flowery bright dress making gazpacho soup in the hot summer days; making a mess in the kitchen baking bread . . . there are so many, many beautiful memories. All of that gave me a strong foundation upon which to build my relationship with food. Not many people today have that in their lives, and that's why so many struggle with weight issues. However, while living away from home as a teenager, processed foods and tons of sugar were slowly introduced into my diet.

During these years I adopted new eating habits. Like so many others, I ate fast food on the run and sugar became the number one ingredient consumed in my diet. I stopped appreciating food, gained a lot of weight and then began dieting, all of which drove my entire body into shock and left my food belief system in shambles. The truth is that most children, teenagers and even adults, are so gullible that they absorb every bit of information (be it right or misleading) they hear and read. This is how each one of us builds what I call your *food belief system* and it soon becomes your reality. Throughout life you continue to look for reinforcement to strengthen these beliefs. This phenomenon is not just limited to food; it happens with everything else in your life as well. However, these beliefs can be changed, even transformed along the way. Let me give you an example.

I grew up in a home with a very positive reinforcement about food, I was always healthy and nobody in my family ever had a weight problem. My reality said that food was something to enjoy and something that also kept me fit and healthy. However, living away from home I adapted a new lifestyle and my eating habits changed dramatically, thus, the unavoidable weight gain. As I struggled to understand what was happening I began inquiring in all the wrong places, asking girlfriends, absorbing weight loss tips from fashion magazines and pouring over fad diet books. This led me to forget about all the wonderful lessons my culture and family instilled in me, and I started listening to the misinformation I thought would give me the results I desired. The more I read the more confused I was and the worse my weight struggle became. I bought into the madness of fad diets and starving myself and, slowly but surely, I began to label food as the enemy.

It wasn't until I finally reached out to reconnect with my culinary roots that I realized how much misinformation and misleading products abound on the shelves of our grocery stores. This sent me on a journey of self-discovery to learn about nutrition and food, with the goal to return to good health and never again struggle with weight or food issues.

Many people use food to justify every situation in their lives. When they're happy, they eat. When they're sad, they eat. When they're depressed and stressed, when they're lonely, when they're in love, when anything major happens to them ... they eat. Soon it seems that with everything they do and feel they simply cannot stop eating. And this is what a person's relationship with food eventually becomes. Eat and then eat some more. Whatever is available or whatever your cravings dictate.

I can relate to this because it was once me. Leaving behind childhood and entering puberty are difficult years in anyone's life, and also very crucial. I spent a large part of those very important years away from home attending school in America. As my diet changed, so did my behavior around food.

When I was sad or missed home, I tried to make myself feel better with sugar and other junk foods that were so widely available because good home cooked meals were absent. Eating sugar and junk became a mechanism to try to feel better, but the sad truth is that these foods only made me feel worse. I was developing self-destructive behaviors rather than nourishing and caring for myself. Unfortunately, this is the type of relationship I developed with food during my teenage years, and it spilled over into my twenties.

After many years of pain and struggle I finally decided to change my point of view about food and certainly about myself, and that's when I began my journey to reconcile with food, my weight and reconnect with my Mediterranean heritage. Once I did that, almost magically, my body and mind became balanced to the point where food has never been a problem again. I enjoy food now as much as when I was growing up in Spain and have no restrictions with regard to what I should and shouldn't eat, as long as what I'm eating is wholesome – not processed – and made with love. And, believe it or not, I have no idea of the caloric content of any of the foods I eat and would never dare to count fats or carbs. It simply doesn't matter.

The major shift that took place in my life was being able to come to terms with food and then consciously choosing to create the healthy friendship I have with it today. Food is no longer something that fills a void. It is no longer cookies and chocolate-covered peanuts while numbing my feelings in front of the TV. Food is wholesome, home cooked meals shared with loved ones; the same way they were cooked at home when I was growing up. And if I happen to be alone, it's just the same. I'm still sharing an amazing home cooked meal with a most loved one, myself.

Cooking raises the awareness of every one of my senses and makes me feel alive. Food is a celebration of life's wonderful gifts and the abundance of the land. Today, no processed foods can ever be found in my pantry because there is no longer any room for junk. That means no snacks with labels screaming "fat free," "low calorie" and all the marketing jargon written on wrappers and boxes that are used to make us buy seemingly "healthy," but nevertheless processed junk foods. Instead, my snacks now consist of natural yogurt with lots of raw cocoa, green tea, crunchy nuts, and combinations of fresh fruits and vegetables. Absolutely yogurtlicious!

Changing your relationship with food is a journey; it doesn't happen from one day to the next, so you better make it a fun and joyous ride. Remember, you'll be enjoying the kinds of foods that can only have a positive effect on you and your health for the rest of your life.

Here, then, are five major steps you must absolutely follow in order to change your relationship with food.

1. **Embrace wholesome food as your ally, not your enemy.** Adopt a positive attitude towards food and everything else will follow.

2. **Search for good quality wholesome ingredients.** Buy fresh produce; skip the frozen, canned and packed food aisles. Eat at restaurants that care more about the food and their guests than quarterly profits.

3. **Think of the kitchen as your sanctuary.** Cooking is a perfect time to disconnect from the world and be with one's self. Focus on nothing else but every detail of the cooking process. Enjoy the peace and time alone. If you have a family, be smart about it and turn it into family time during which everyone part takes in the process. Don't forget to include the kids so that they start building a strong and healthy relationship with food from an early age.

4. **Cook homemade meals with love.** Love is the most important ingredient in your pantry.

5. **Have fun in the kitchen.** Chose ingredients and recipes that are delicious and that you enjoy making.

Foods You *Cannot* Eat
On the Yogurt Diet

The Yogurt Diet is quite simple. The foods you must avoid are foods that contain yeasts or foods that feed yeasts and parasites. These include ALL processed foods; any foods that contain yeasts, such as wine and beer, bread, moldy and aged cheeses, vinegar, and pickled foods with vinegar; mushrooms, because they are a fungi (yeasts are also a fungi); sugar, and anything containing sugar because yeast and parasites love sugar; wheat, and anything containing wheat, such as breads, pasta, cookies; bottled juices and artificial sweeteners. Sounds quite simple and easy, right? The truth is that it should be. However, these are precisely the foods you most likely crave and normally eat everyday of your life. So at first it will be challenging to break these patterns. You'll probably begin to think there is nothing for you to eat anymore, but soon after you begin following the Yogurt Diet your cravings will disappear and it will become easier and easier to adhere to the program.

Fruits are some of the healthiest foods the land has to offer, they're full of vitamins, minerals, enzymes, fiber and antioxidants. But during the Yogurt Diet there is one non-negotiable rule you must follow when it comes to eating fruits. **Always eat fruits with yogurt.** Here's why. Fruits are rich in the sugar fructose, and yeasts love this type of sugar. But so do healthy bacteria that abound in yogurt. When you combine fruit with yogurt, it is the good bacteria that get to the sugars first. This prevents yeasts and other harmful guys from getting to them and causing weight and health problems.

When you have an overgrowth of yeast in your body and you eat fruit without yogurt, the yeast devours the fructose and ferments the sugars in your belly producing alcohol, carbon dioxide and a list of toxins that can enter your bloodstream. Not to mention the fact that you continue feeding this monster, which keeps growing, making you fat and producing toxins that lead to many diseases. You must also remember that not all fruits are created equal. Some of the fruits you cannot eat during the Yogurt Diet are those with very high sugar content (all types of melons, pineapple and figs) or those very high in yeasts, such as all berries, plums and grapes. All other fruits that have a skin must be rinsed well under running water and *always* be combined with yogurt. Needless to say, avoid bottled juices at all times. This is non negotiable, no matter how healthy the label promotes it to be. You should always drink fruit juices fresh, not pasteurized and not bottled stored on shelves for days and even weeks. Drink water whenever you're thirsty. In fact, drink plenty of water every day of your life, to nourish every cell and organ in your body and help in the cleansing process.

Not All Milk Products are Created Equal

There are two criteria that you need to look for when choosing dairy products while following the Yogurt Diet.

1. Has the milk product been fermented with lactic acid bacteria or "live cultures?" Such is the case with yogurt, kefir and butter.

2. What types of microorganisms are present? This is very important, because aged and moldy cheeses contain yeasts and molds in them, which do not make these dairy products appropriate to eat during the detoxifying process intended with the Yogurt Diet.

Because your body is in a state of imbalance, moldy cheeses will continue to harm you and defeat the goal you're trying to reach. Remember, this doesn't mean that these types of cheeses are unhealthy, only under the condition of an imbalanced bacterial flora can and do they cause harm. When following the Yogurt Diet, stick to probiotic yogurt, kefir and butter to avoid confusion when you're working toward bringing your body back into harmony. Once this is achieved, you will once again be able to enjoy the wide spectrum of delicious dairy products without ever worrying about weight gain or intolerances.

Food Foes

Sugar and high fructose corn syrup
Always check labels.

Fruits
Watermelon, honeydew, cantaloupe, grapes, pineapple, figs, plums.

Berries
Strawberries, blueberries, blackberries, raspberries, boysenberries, etc. These fruits have very porous skins where yeasts live. Even after washing, yeasts still remain in the pores of the fruit.

Jams and jellies
All kinds, even those claiming to have no sugar added.

Bottled fruit and vegetable juices
Found in the super-market, even if they are orgainic. Make your own at home —fresh—and drink right away.

Dried, canned and candied fruits
Raisins, apricots, figs, prunes, peaches, blueberries, pineapple, banana, dates, etc.

Malt products
Found mostly in cereals, sodas and candy.

Sodas
All kinds.

Packaged and processed foods
Canned, bottled and boxed foods most likely contain sugar, HSCF and other hidden ingredients.

Potatoes
None of any kind.

Food Foes

White Rice
And pre-cooked packaged rice containing flavors and spices.

Baked goods
Bread, pastries, tortillas and other flat breads,
crackers, cereals, cookies.

Wheat
All wheat products, such as whole wheat, white flour, kamut,
wheat berries, spelt, semolina, and wheat couscous.
Also barley and rye. These grains are found in cereals, breads,
baked goods, pasta and alcoholic beverages, among other foods.

Dairy
Pasteurized milk. Aged and moldy cheeses, which are
easily identified because they have an outer crust. Stay away from
commercially made sour cream, buttermilk, and yogurts with
sugar, fruits, citric acid and preservatives.

Fish
No farm raised. No sushi.

Alcoholic beverages
All of them, such as beer, wine and hard liquor.

Vinegar
And all condiments containing vinegar such as
mustard, ketchup, mayonnaise, salad dressings, pickled
vegetables etc. Check labels.

Mushrooms
All types.

Soy products
Including soy sauce, soymilk, tofu and bean curd.

Food Foes

Processed and smoked meats and fish
Cold cuts, sausage, hot dogs, smoked salmon, smoked meats, beef jerky, pastrami, etc.

Oils
Soy, corn, sunflower, safflower, peanut; low fat and non-stick oil sprays; all hydrogenated oils, including margarines, Crisco and cake frostings.

Pickled foods
All pickled vegetables containing sugar, vinegar, acetic acid or preservatives among the ingredients. Check labels.

Vegetables
Canned, bottled and overcooked vegetables.

Corn
Is a grain, not a vegetable. Avoid all its byproducts.

Coffee and Tea
Many coffees and teas contain molds. Be cautious to buy high quality teas. Stay away from coffee. No kombucha tea.

Herbs
Irradiated herbs.

Salt
Avoid processed salts, such as iodized salts.

Leftovers
Molds grow on leftovers that are not refrigerated right away. It's better to freeze food if you cook to last for a few days. Reheat slowly on the stove until reaching boiling point (around 210 F). Avoid microwaving.

Foods You *Can* Eat
On the Yogurt Diet

You can eat everything else, all fresh vegetables and fruits on the list – seeds and nuts, vegetables which have been naturally fermented with LAB, fish, meat, chicken, lamb, goat, rabbit, duck, dried beans and all grains that do not contain wheat; agave (the most delectable sweetener), coconut oil and plenty of extra virgin olive oil and, of course, yogurt and more yogurt, and also kefir. That's quite a variety of good foods.

Aside from the food list, there are two simple rules to follow:

1. Always combine raw vegetables along with cooked vegetables with every meal for life and active enzymes. Cooked vegetables are also necessary, as in many instances some nutrients are enhanced during the cooking process.

2. Always eat fruit with yogurt.

Food Allys

Vegetables
All green, white and colorful vegetables; also root vegetables such as beets, carrots, jicama, radish; and bulb vegetables, including onions, shallots and garlic; all squash varieties. Eat them cooked and raw.

Fruits
Apples, bananas, oranges, lemons, mangos, pears, kiwis, coconuts, tangerines, apricots, peaches, nectarines, kumquats, cherries, cherimoya, pomegranate. Wash them well and always eat with yogurt.

Beans
All varieties of dried beans. Cook them at home.
Do not buy canned.

Food Allys

Meat and eggs
Free range, humanly treated, free of antibiotics and hormones.
These include beef, chicken, turkey, lamb, pork, eggs, rabbit,
bison, venison, etc.

Fish
Fish should always be wild caught and fresh. Eat a variety of smaller
fish. You may eat raw fish with lots of lemon or lime.

Nuts and seeds
Assorted raw nuts and seeds: macadamia, pistachios, pine, Brazil,
almonds, hazelnuts, walnuts, sesame, sunflower, pumpkin, flax etc.

Oils
ONLY cold pressed oils, such as extra virgin olive oil, coconut oil and
coconut butter, sesame oil, nut oils (except peanut oil), flax seed and
avocado oil.

Dairy
Natural yogurt, kefir and butter with live active cultures.

Grains
Oats, amaranth, whole grain rice (all varieties), quinoa, millet and
buckwheat (not a wheat grain). The rule is whole grain varieties
without wheat and gluten.

Herbs and Spices
Fresh and dried organic herbs and spices

Salt
Sea salt, Himalayan pink salt. All natural salts.

Others
Agave (a natural sweetener), probiotics (active bacteria), pollen,
Pao D'Arco tea, matcha green tea and raw cocoa.

Three Meals a Day

The Yogurt Diet recommends that you eat three times a day. I personally don't believe in one of the latest fads, which recommends that you eat six or more small meals a day. People who follow this rule tend to under eat throughout the day, only to come home at night and raid the pantry and/or refrigerator. In all honesty, I'm sorry to be the one breaking this news to you, but a handful of nuts or a cheese stick is not a meal by any means. Traditional cultures eat three meals a day. This has been the case for many, many years, and I certainly tend to adhere to this proven rule. There's no need to reinvent the wheel here. It seems we have fared pretty well doing this in the past. Better yet, there's a scientific explanation of why you should eat three normal meals a day, rather than six "birdie" meals.

Having fewer meals a day is beneficial for the body's health and to maintain normal weight. Frequent eating and snacking puts added pressure on your digestive system and decreases enzyme levels, leading to weight gain. The organs involved in digestion need to rest, and suffer greatly when you don't allow them a break. Experiments have shown that animals fed fewer times a day lived almost 20 percent longer, were slimmer and had more enzyme activity in their pancreas and fat cells. Their counterparts, who ate more often, developed more fat cells in the body. This is the same reaction seen in overfed children who develop obesity.

The three meals you should be eating during the day are breakfast, lunch and dinner. The Yogurt Diet recommends enough food at each meal so that you don't crave snacks between meals. When you sit down to eat, you should eat wholesome foods to your satisfaction. Regardless of what you may have heard before, don't leave the table feeling hungry. The purpose of eating a meal is to feel fulfilled. Of course, don't misconstrue this recommendation and think that it's okay to gorge. That is not acceptable. Portion control is extremely important.

There are some other reasons why you should eat three meals a day. Here's what each one does for you.

Breakfast – Jumpstarts your metabolism in the morning. The word breakfast literally means "to break the fast," and it does just that. It breaks the fasting period that your body has undergone since you ate dinner the evening before. Without breakfast your body is sluggish because it perceives that it is still in fasting mode. When this happens, your body retains energy, accumulates fat, burns enzyme stores and doesn't get the engines running at full speed. That's why it is so important to honor this first meal of the day. At the same time, because breakfast is breaking a fast of many hours, your body is at rest and not ready to start digesting a big breakfast composed of heavily cooked foods. Instead, start your day with enzyme, antioxidant, vitamin, mineral and probiotic rich foods also high in fiber. The Yogurt Diet recommends that you start your day with a combination of yogurt and other raw ingredients, as well as a serving of grain of your choice. This is the breakfast of champions, full of probiotic bacteria and enzymes, rich in health and youth promoting nutrients, and packed with fiber. No doubt this combination of foods will rev up your metabolism and start your engines running at full speed from the moment you get up, ensuring that you're well on your way to a speedy weight loss and the restoration of your health.

Lunch – During the day you're burning fuel like crazy. Your metabolism is in fifth gear so that you can function optimally, with super energy and focus. However, the burned fuel must be restocked, because if it's not, your metabolism will slow down in order to conserve the energy that's not being replaced. If you skip lunch in order to eat fewer calories or you tell yourself that you're too busy to care enough for your wellbeing, you'll ultimately be hurting your health and have a more difficult time finding your ideal weight. When you skip lunch, you work up such hunger that your energy level will slow down. You will ultimately surrender to eating what ever comes your way at work, usually something in the form of sugar. Then, on your way home you will stop at the window of some horrific fast food joint to pick up dinner. In your famished condition, the idea of stopping at the supermarket and making a homemade meal is nearly unfathomable. This is a perpetual self-defeating cycle, one that will have you wondering why you can't stick to your diet plan and why you never feel your best. There's good reason why there's lunch in the middle of the day. Honor this meal and never skip it.

Dinner – This, in my opinion, is the most enjoyable meal of the day. Dinner is really a time to celebrate — celebrate life, celebrate magnificent food and share your day and dreams around a beautiful table with loved ones. It is a time when you can unwind and let go of all the stress of the day, a time to get close to loved ones, laugh and enjoy life. Why would any one want to skip this most enjoyable of meals? There's also far more to dinner than you might think. Remember, you've had a busy day running around, burning fuel, and this naturally depletes your body of nutrients, exposes your body to many toxins and microbes, and oxidizes cells. All this wear and tear must be restored. Also, dinner is the last meal of the day before you go to sleep for an overnight fast. While you sleep your body goes through a detoxification and replenishing process, and it needs all the help it can get. Dinner is the meal to fill up with nutritious foods that will help repair every cell in your body while you sleep. This important event needs plenty of energy; so don't be afraid to eat a healthful meal two to four hours before going to bed. Your metabolism doesn't stop just because you stop. Be smart and eat your three meals a day for your metabolism to keep running twenty-four/seven. Having nourishment in your system before going to sleep ensures that you have a good night's rest. You will have a difficult time going to sleep on an empty stomach, and when you don't sleep properly weight gain can begin to creep up on your bones. Needless to say, never skip dinner.

In addition, never question skipping a meal for the sake of saving calories, because the eventual bill for doing that will be passed on to you with a huge interest. In other words, you'll ultimately pay. The more rigorous you are about eating a nutritious and fulfilling breakfast, lunch and dinner, the easier weight loss becomes.

Food Combinations —
The Two-Course Meal

This is a very important aspect of the Yogurt Diet, because developing a balanced body is highly dependent on eating foods in the best order and in combinations that will assist in better digestion as well as aiding your body in assimilating nutrients while getting your metabolism jump-started.

Remember, your body is not sustained by what you eat but rather by what it absorbs. For the body to fully take in all nutrients and achieve complete digestion it needs the two major drivers — probiotic bacteria and enzymes — which make sure that nutrients can be properly digested and absorbed into the blood stream. Without these two essential components digestion will be poor, nutrients will not be absorbed and the downward spiral to bad health will begin, resulting in an out of balance body taxed with food intolerances, weight gain and disease.

Both digestion and metabolism are maintained by enzyme activity. If your body lacks enzymes or the foods you eat lack enzymes, your health and weight will suffer to varying degrees. To bring your enzymes levels back you need to start consuming lots of yogurt and raw foods.

Whole milk yogurt contains the wide spectrum of essential nutrients: carbohydrates, proteins and fats. Not surprisingly, many of the enzymes present in yogurt are the same type needed by your body to break down carbohydrates, proteins and fats present in other foods. The fat portion in milk is important, because if you eat fat free yogurt you will fail to replenish essential enzymes that are crucial for the metabolism of fats in your body. For this reason, you should always consume whole milk yogurt with live active bacteria if you want to lose weight. People living in Mediterranean countries consume their yogurt in its wholeness, even sometimes adding extra cream to make it luxuriously rich. These people are not overweight, nor do they suffer from coronary disease. That's because, contrary to what we have been led to believe, the fat in milk does not make you fat. This is a widespread misconception that needs to be corrected. Millions of thin and healthy people will attest that eating fat from milk products is healthy and does not contribute to weight gain. It is an individual's imbalances that are to blame.

Whole yogurt is one of the few existing foods containing the enzymes which can break down all the nutrients — proteins, fats and carbohydrates. This makes yogurt a perfect food to add to your meals as it can, among other things, act as an enzyme and bacterial boost. By contrast, most other foods only have enzymes that can metabolize fats, carbohydrates or proteins individually, but not all at once. The enzymes in yogurt, however, can. That's why I call yogurt the "Microbe and Enzyme Cocktail." All foods also contain specific enzymes that will assist in their own metabolism, so it is important to always add some raw and not highly processed foods to your every meal.

The Yogurt Diet is based on a *two-course meal* approach. You will always start both lunch and dinner with a soup or vegetable-based salad, followed by a main course of equal portions of protein, vegetables and grains. There are three important reasons to start your meal always with a soup or salad. One, you will eat less; two, you will have a more nutritious and balanced meal; and three, your digestion and metabolism will work at peak performance using this method.

Eating your veggies first is a good technique to prevent you from overeating. Fruits and vegetables are light and easy to digest because of their high water content (90-97 percent), and they're also very high in fiber and nutrients, which makes them filling when you eat them. Fiber rich foods create bulk and fill you up, thus preventing you from overeating. They also aid in digestion by helping your digestive system to speed up transit time, while also feeding your bacterial flora. Starting a meal with vegetables is a good practice because it prevents you from eating a one pound steak or a huge bowl of pasta. The other side of the coin is that by the time your second course arrives — with protein, more vegetables and grains — your initial hunger will have subsided and four ounces of chicken will look just the prefect size. By the time you're done with your nutritious and fulfilling two-course meal, the dessert cart will be out of the question. This is one of the tricks and nutritional practices followed in traditional diets. Meals are comprised of various courses, most times starting with a vegetable dish.

The purpose of eating a two-course meal is also for you to take in all the nutrients your body needs with a smart variety of foods — plenty of vegetables, just the right amount of protein and fat, and the right portion of grains — so that you feel satisfied, rather than feeling constant hunger and the need to be snacking. When you eat a two-course meal, you also combine flavors and textures, keeping it more exciting with variation. And when you sit down to eat, EAT! Do it with joy and pleasure, take your time and then put it behind you. This way food will not take up the bulk of your thoughts throughout the day, taking away from other activities that demand your total concentration. You will become a lot more productive and your boss will love you, and you will also have more time to do the things you love.

Always combine raw and cooked vegetables with your meals. If you have a soup for your first course, then eat a salad with the main course. And if you chose to eat the salad first, then have a tomato sauce, sautéed or steamed vegetables with your main meal.

Portion Size

This is what I call, **"Eat to Your Hand Size."** Put your hand up in front of you and check it out carefully, as if this was the very first time you're seeing it. How big is your hand? Is it very big, big, medium or small? Next, spread your fingers open and bend them over slightly. Do you see the scoop you've formed with your hand? Look at it and imagine food in it. That's exactly the perfect portion size for you. No more, no less. That's literally what's commonly known as a hand full. You will be using this simple method to measure portions during the Yogurt Diet and beyond. In fact, you can use it for the rest of your life. Remember, you'll be eating a two-course meal, so you'll have to repeat this process with each serving on your plate.

Let's say you're having a salad for your first course. Whatever fits in your slightly bent hand is how big your salad should be. Add a variety of vegetables, nuts or yogurt of your choice, but always using your hand as a guide, for yourself and for other people if you're cooking for them. Notice that most salads have greens, or other vegetables that are fluffy in nature.

When making soup, this measurement technique works much the same. How much soup can fit in your bent hand? (This is just an approximation. You obviously can't serve soup with your hand.) That's how much soup should be in your bowl. To give you an idea, it will be about 1 1/2-2 cups. Pretty easy, right? No measuring tools and no scales are required, just your hand. This makes life so much easier.

Now it's time for the main course. Again, put your hand up in front of you, only this time bring your fingers closely together and bend them over. You will notice that the scoop of your hand has become smaller. That's exactly the portion of vegetables, grains and protein you may enjoy to the fullest on your main course. So, to build a main course, add a handful of raw or cooked vegetables, a handful of cooked grains and a handful of protein.

You will soon realize that eating "for your hand size" keeps you absolutely satisfied and always in control. This method simply never fails. It's also a great way to teach children about portion size, something they will remember for the rest of their lives.

Let's say you're 5'6" tall. You will need about four ounces of protein at one meal. Keep in mind that you will also be eating yogurt, which is also part of your protein intake. On the other hand, if you're six feet tall and well built your hands will be larger and you should eat accordingly. You might need up to six ounces of chicken, plus a serving of the recommended yogurt with your meal.

Surprisingly, servings in the Yogurt Diet are quite generous so that you never feel hungry. Eat slowly, enjoy every bite, and if you can't finish everything on your plate that's okay as long as you feel satisfied.

Rampant snacking is not allowed during the Yogurt Diet. However, many people do enjoy eating their yogurt treats before or after lunch or dinner, rather than right after their meal. This is quite acceptable. So eat your yogurt desserts whenever you please, just as long as you eat three servings of yogurt a day.

About Exercise

Exercise is essential during all stages of one's life. It can be anything from a walk in the park, playing golf or basketball, jogging, sprinting, climbing up stairs or lifting weights. But the most important thing about exercise is that you find something you love and will look forward to doing. Personally, I am not much of a gym rat. I like being outdoors jogging or playing tennis and enjoying the beautiful sun while I get a dose of vitamin D. People generally think that I exercise a lot or I couldn't possibly be my size with the amount of food I eat. Or people say that I'm lucky because I was born with a fast metabolism. I exercise to have fun and yes, I was born with a fast metabolism just like everyone else. But I also had two choices: one, to slow down my fast metabolism; or two, to continue feeding the engine that keeps that metabolism running as fast as a Lamborghini Diablo.

My advice is to find an activity you like doing and go for at least thirty minutes, ideally up to an hour, four days a week. The purpose is not to burn calories, but rather to move your body because the benefits are endless. Buy a racket and find a playing partner. You don't have to be a pro. You'll get enough exercise just running after the ball. And the best thing is that it's fun. All you need is to work up a sweat so you can eliminate toxins circulating in your body. That, and having fun, should be your major concerns, not burning calories.

Take a Sauna

If you have access to a sauna, go for it. This is also a superb way to eliminate toxic waste through the pores of your skin. You need to keep those elimination organs as stimulated and clean as possible. However, if you don't have access to a sauna, buy a loofa glove or bath brush and brush off dead cells from the body using upward circular motions. This also gets your lymph system moving and, again, helps remove toxins.

A Final Conclusion

The Yogurt diet is the delicious and fulfilling way of eating without ever having to worry about calories, fats and carbs. You simply have to adhere to a list of foods and combine them properly to create magnificent meals. That's it! Nothing fancy, nothing exotic. The most important by-product of the Yogurt Diet is bringing your life into harmony. The end result is ideal weight, phenomenal health, radiant beauty, unstoppable energy and a positive outlook on life.

Even though there are some restrictions as to the foods you can eat, the goal of the Yogurt diet is loud and clear. **Cleanse your body and put it in a state of balance so that you will be able to enjoy all the foods you love once again.**

The most interesting change you'll see after following the Yogurt Diet is that, when your body is finally in harmony, many of the foods you craved or enjoyed before will lose their attraction and even taste awful. In fact, you'll probably wonder how you ate them for so long. From that point on you will have become a conscious eater and you will seek only the most wholesome foods and the best ingredients possible.

The best news? You will finally have won the battle against disease, uncontrollable cravings and unattractive weight gain. And, thanks to the Yogurt Diet, it will be a permanent victory.

Salud!

Chapter Seven

Let's Start Cooking

Our lives are not in the lap of the gods, but in the lap of our cooks.

— Lin Yutang (Chinese writer)

The recipes that follow in this chapter are easy and fun to make. Begin by stacking your refrigerator and pantry with the ingredients you will need for the recipes of the week. It's much easier to find all the ingredients under one roof, especially if you do your grocery shopping at a health supermarket that carries plenty of wholesome foods and where the employees will graciously help you find all the ingredients you need. Once you become proficient at this first step you'll see how easy it becomes making permanent changes to your lifestyle.

Remember Rome was not built in a day. Take one step at a time and always acknowledge yourself with love and encouragement for the positive changes you make. Just know that each day you're following the Yogurt Diet you're that much closer to having a balanced body and achieving your goals for ultimate health and weight.

A Tip or Two to Start on the Right Foot

Breakfast – We all have places to go, people to see and new worlds to conquer every morning. There's often no time to fuss around breakfast and that's why the Yogurt Diet is totally uncomplicated, quick and easy. Breakfast is all about giving your body that initial morning boost it needs to jumpstart your day.

Because I wanted to save the best for last, I have a delicious surprise for you that I've been eager to tell you all along. Are you ready? How would you like it if I tell you that all throughout the Yogurt Diet you must start your day with a big bowl of "yogurtlicious" chocolate or green tea yogurt. That's right, I'm not kidding! Wow, can life get any better than that? Indeed, this is great news for dieters who often feel deprived from enjoying their favorite foods. Not on the Yogurt Diet, instead, this is a must.

So each morning from here on, you will start your day with one of the jazzy raw cocoa or matcha green tea yogurt recipes in the **smoothies and desserts section** of this chapter. Here's why. Raw cocoa and matcha green tea are two super power foods that, when mixed with yogurt, become a health dynamite cocktail. And I mean this literally, because this combination of foods is an explosion of energy, antioxidants, vitamins, minerals, enzymes, probiotics and prebiotics.

Raw cocoa is the purest form of what we commonly know as chocolate. The heavenly pleasure of eating raw cocoa with abandon is something to celebrate and not feel guilty about. This super food contains many naturally occurring chemicals that enhance mental and physical wellbeing, and it contains way more antioxidant flavanoids than red wine and blueberries. These antioxidants are known to help maintain healthy blood flow and blood pressure, which promote cardiovascular health; as well as having anti-aging and anti-inflammatory properties. With this long list of health benefits don't be surprised when I tell you that before cocoa is brought to your table it goes trough a process of fermentation by various probiotic organisms. Indeed, some of the same lactic acid bacteria present in the fermentation of milk that turns it into yogurt is also responsible for cocoa fermentation. No wonder it's so healthy.

Matcha green tea is the best quality green tea available and it's also super rich in the antioxidants flavanoids, with 200 times the antioxidant levels of normal green tea. Rich in theanine (vitamin B1), it increases the alpha wave activity in the brain to enhance relaxation and focus. Matcha green tea improves blood flow, helps eliminate toxins, and boosts the immune system. This super tea protects against cardiovascular disease and has anti-microbial, anti-carcinogenic and anti-inflammatory powers. Among the newest benefits found in matcha green tea is the effectiveness in speeding metabolism and aiding in weight loss.

That said, you should start your day with a raw cocoa or matcha green tea yogurt dynamite cocktail every morning. Okay, now you're half way there. Then, while you're picking your snazziest outfit and shoes to match, put your oatmeal or another grain to cook on the stove. And before you even have a chance to tighten your belt buckle to keep your pants on your newfound waist, your oatmeal will be ready to go. Easy breezy!

Remember, in the **smoothies and dessert section** of this chapter you'll find a great number of quick and easy ways to make yogurt recipes using a combination of delicious and super nutritious fruits and vegetables, nuts, raw cocoa, coconut butter, matcha green tea and other ingredients. The palate pleasing result will be smoothies and frozen yogurt treats that you can eat for breakfast or at any other time of the day.

Antioxidants

Antioxidants are closely correlated in the prevention of cellular damage – a common cause for aging, cancer, and a list of other diseases. Antioxidants are molecules that safely interact with free radicals and terminate the chain reaction before damage can occur to molecules that are vital for life. This is essentially one of the major jobs of vitamin C in the body. There are several enzyme systems within the body that scavenge free radicals, but the main antioxidants are vitamin E, beta-carotene (Vitamin A), and vitamin C. Because the body cannot manufacture these micronutrients they must be supplied in the diet.

Lunch – Most of us eat lunch at work. The best advice is to take your time and don't rush. Every company should enforce this practice for the simple reason that people become more productive when their minds have rested for an hour and they have eaten a nutritious meal. Since we eat lunch at work, we also need to be prepared to fulfill the needs of the Yogurt Diet. Remember that eating a small salad with fat-free dressing will simply not cut it. This is not the essence of the Yogurt Diet. You must eat a two-course meal, starting with a soup or salad, followed by a main course with a good source of protein, more vegetables and a wholesome grain, plus a yogurt treat. This is extremely important while you're following this diet.

Remember, there's very good reason for the two-course meal. Whether you bring your lunch from home or eat at a restaurant, this formula must be followed. And always have yogurt handy, stacked in your office's refrigerator or in a cooler you keep in the car. The idea is to eat enough healthy foods so that you will never succumb to sugar cravings in late afternoon.

Dinner – The best meal of the day, indeed. Dinner is the one meal during which you can fully practice creating a new relationship with food because you should have the necessary time to invest in cooking, not to mention truly enjoying eating the marvelous foods you have prepared. This doesn't mean that your entire evening should be about cooking. The recipes that follow are easy and not too time consuming. And you will notice that as you grow into a more avid cook, you will also become more skillful and time efficient. Making a two-course meal will be something you'll really look forward to. What the Yogurt Diet recommends is that you always make a little extra food for dinner so that you can have extra to eat for lunch the next day and save you time from having to cook too many meals in a day. But if you're like me, then you might want to cook a fresh dish for every meal. Now, let's start cooking!

5-Week Meal Plan

Three Days of Bacteria and Enzyme Super Boost

The first three days of the Yogurt Diet are an initial boost to get your system mobilizing to drive the toxins – which have accumulated for so many years – out of your body. This is a gentle way to start bringing your body back into harmony.

To do this, the menus for days one, two and three are based on raw foods and lots of yogurt. When eaten together they will give you the enzyme and bacteria boost your body needs to start this cleansing and restoring process. Be aware that the "not so pleasant" symptoms you may experience are due to the sewer system finally getting unplugged. Write down everything you're experiencing each day in a journal so that you can keep it for your records. This is very important.

Day 1

Breakfast

Matcha green tea yogurt of your choice (page 302-304)

add 2 tablespoons raw pistachios

Lunch

Soup: Cucumber soup (page 256)

Main: Coleslaw with raw pumpkin seeds (page 242)

Yogurt Dessert

Cocoa coconut crunch frozen yogurt (page 298)

Dinner

Main: Maché and raw beet salad (page 229)

Yogurt Dessert

Yogurt dessert of your choice (page 288-304)

Day 2

Breakfast
Cocoa Mono Loco smoothie (page 301)

Lunch
Main: Greek salad with (page 243)

Yogurt Dessert
Rose water almond yogurt (page 294)

Dinner
Soup: Gazpacho (page 249)

Main: Caesar salad with raw pumpkin seeds (page 228)

Yogurt Dessert
Cucumber smoothie of your choice (page 295-297)

Day 3

Breakfast

Matcha green tea yogurt of your choice (pages 302-304)

add 1 tablespoon raw almonds

Lunch

Salad: Tomato cucumber kefir salad (page 227)

Main: Thai tuna carpaccio (page 213)

with mango chutney (page 278)

Yogurt Dessert

Yogurt dessert of your choice (pages 288-304)

Dinner

Salad: Very summery salad (page 235)

Main: Ceviche of monkfish (page 221)

with guacamole (page 276)

Yogurt Dessert

Totally orange smoothie (page 293)

To make the transition easy on your digestive system after eating an all-raw foods diet for three days, start day four by eating a vegetarian diet with plenty of vegetables and the addition of cooked starches.

Breakfast

Raw cocoa yogurt of your choice (page 298-301)

Grain: Natural organic oatmeal (page 271)

(or whole grain of your choice) (page 259)

Lunch

Salad: Very summery salad with (page 235)

Main: Ceviche of monkfish (page 221)

with guacamole (page 276)

Yogurt Dessert

Lassi (page 290)

Dinner

Soup: Red lentil soup (page 246)

Grain/main: Couscous salad (page 265)

Yogurt Dessert

Cucumber apple and celery smoothie (page 296)

Day 5

Breakfast

Matcha green tea yogurt of your choice (page 302-304)

Grain: Natural organic oatmeal (page 271)

(or whole grain of your choice) (page 259)

Lunch

Soup: Red lentil soup (page 246)

Grain/main: Couscous salad (page 265)

Yogurt Dessert

Mango orange yogurt smoothie (page 292)

Dinner

Yogurt Drink: Lassi (page 290)

Salad: New York salad (page 233)

Main: Pisto with fried eggs (page 206)

Grain: Short grain rice   (page 259)

Breakfast

Raw cocoa yogurt of your choice (page 298-301)

Grain: Natural organic oatmeal (page 271)

(or whole grain of your choice) (page 259)

Lunch

Yogurt Drink: Cucumber kiwi lime smoothie (page 297)

Salad: New York salad (page 233)

Main: Pisto with soft-cooked eggs (page 206)

Grain: Short grain rice (page 259)

Dinner

Salad: Caesar salad (page 228)

Main/Starch: White bean stew and scallops (page 203)

Yogurt Dessert

Yogurt dessert of your choice (page 288-304)

*Note: fried eggs taste best when cooked on the spot and eaten right away. In this lunch recipe, if you're taking the food to go from the previous night's dinner, it's best to eat this dish with soft-cooked eggs (page 202) instead.

Day 7

Breakfast

Matcha green tea yogurt of your choice (page 302-304)

Grain: Natural organic oatmeal (page 271)

(or whole grain of your choice) (page 259)

Lunch

Salad: Caesar salad (page 228)

Main/ complex starch: White bean stew and scallops (page 203)

Yogurt Dessert

Yogurt and fresh fruit with raw macadamia nuts (page 289)

Dinner

Soup: Gazpacho (page 249)

Main: Super chicken salad (page 197)

Grain: Red quinoa (page 259)

Yogurt Dessert

Yogurt dessert of your choice (page 288-304)

Day 8

Breakfast

Raw cocoa yogurt of your choice (page 298-301)

Grain: Natural organic oatmeal (page 271)

(or whole grain of your choice) (page 259)

Lunch

Soup: Gazpacho (page 249)

Main: Super chicken salad (page 197)

Grain: Red quinoa (page 259)

Yogurt Dessert

Yogurt dessert of your choice (page 288-304)

Dinner

Salad: Very summery salad (page 235)

Main: Salmon with sweet roasted pepper sauce (page 212)

Grain: Black Rice (page 259)

Yogurt Dessert

Totally orange smoothie (page 293)

Day 9

Breakfast

Matcha green tea yogurt of your choice (page 302-304)

Grain: Natural organic oatmeal (page 271)

(or whole grain of your choice) (page 259)

Lunch

Salad: Very summery salad (page 235)

Main: Salmon with sweet roasted pepper sauce (page 212)

Grain: Black Rice (page 259)

Yogurt Dessert

Rose water almond yogurt (page 294)

Dinner

Salad: Maché and beet salad (page 229)

Main: Peruvian style chicken (page 215)

Grain: Long grain basmati rice (page 259)

Day 10

Breakfast

Raw cocoa yogurt of your choice (page 298-301)

Grain: Natural organic oatmeal (page 271)

(or whole grain of your choice) (page 259)

Lunch

Salad: Maché and beet salad (page 229)

Main: Peruvian style chicken (page 215)

Grain: Long grain basmati rice (page 259)

Dinner

Salad: Tossed salad

Main: Beef stew (page 201)

Grain/ Complex starch: Black lentils (page 258)

Yogurt Dessert

Yogurt dessert of your choice (page 288-304)

Day 11

Breakfast

Matcha green tea yogurt of your choice (page 302-304)

Grain: Natural organic oatmeal (page 271)

(or whole grain of your choice) (page 259)

Lunch

Salad: Tossed salad

Main: Beef stew (page 201)

Grain/ Complex starch: Black lentils (page 258)

Yogurt Dessert

Yogurt dessert of your choice (page 288-304)

Dinner (Vegetarian)

Salad/Complex starch: Humus with vegetables (page 270)

Main/Grain: Quinoa pilaf with red and yellow peppers (Page 264)

and spinach raita (page 239)

Day 12

Breakfast

Raw cocoa yogurt of your choice (page 298-301)

Grain: Natural organic oatmeal (page 271)

(or whole grain of your choice) (page 259)

Lunch

Salad/Complex starch: Humus with vegetables (page 270)

Main/Grain: Quinoa piliaf with red and yeloow peppers (page 264)

and spinach raita (page 239)

Dinner

Soup & starch: Butternut squash soup (page 250)

Main: Crab salad (page 210)

Yogurt Dessert

Yogurt dessert of your choice (page 288-304)

Day 13

Breakfast

Matcha green tea yogurt of your choice (page 302-304)

Grain: Natural organic oatmeal (page 271)

(or whole grain of your choice) (page 259)

Lunch

Soup & starch: Butternut squash soup (page 250)

Main: Crab salad (page 210)

Yogurt Dessert

Yogurt dessert of your choice (page 288-304)

Dinner

Salad: Tossed salad with avocado

Main: Tandoori chcicken with spinach raita   (page 222)

Grain: Brown jasmine rice (page 259)

Yogurt Dessert

Rosewater almond yogurt (page 294)

Day 14

Breakfast

Raw cocoa yogurt of your choice (page 298-301)

Grain: Natural organic oatmeal (page 271)

(or whole grain of your choice) (page 259)

Lunch

Salad: Tossed salad with avocado

Main: Tandoori chcicken with spinach raita (page 222)

Grain: Brown jasmine rice (page 259)

Yogurt Dessert

Totally orange smoothie (page 293)

Dinner

Soup: Carrot soup (page 245)

Yogurt drink: Lassi (page 290)

Main: Sea bass with mango salad (page 298)

Grain: Coconut rice (page 260)

Day 15

Breakfast

Matcha green tea yogurt of your choice (page 302-304)

Grain: Natural organic oatmeal (Page 271)

(or whole grain of your choice) (Page 259)

Lunch

Soup: Carrot soup (page 245)

Yogurt drink: Lassi (page 290)

Main: Sea bass with mango salad (page 298)

Grain: Coconut rice (page 260)

Dinner

Salad: Greek salad (page 243)

Main: Minced meat with tomatoes and eggplant (page 216)

Grain: Basmati wild rice pilaf (page 263)

Day 16

Breakfast

Raw cocoa yogurt of your choice (page 298-301)

Grain: Natural organic oatmeal (page 271)

(or whole grain of your choice) (page 259)

Lunch

Salad: Greek salad (page 243)

Main: Minced meat with tomatoes and eggplant (page 216)

Grain: Basmati wild rice pilaf (page 263)

Dinner

Soup: Gazpacho (page 249)

Main: Oven roasted chicken with roasted vegetables (page 208)

Complex starch: Butternut squash

Yogurt Dessert

Yogurt dessert of your choice (page 288-304)

Day 17

Breakfast

Matcha green tea yogurt of your choice (page 302-304)

Grain: Natural organic oatmeal (page 271)

(or whole grain of your choice) (page 259)

Lunch

Soup: Gazpacho (page 249)

Main: Oven roasted chicken with roasted vegetables (page 208)

Complex starch: Butternut squash

Yogurt Dessert

Cucumber apple and celery smoothie (page 296)

Dinner

Salad: Very summery salad (page 235)

Main: Thai chicken soup (page 257)

Grain: Short grain coconut rice   (page 260)

Yogurt Dessert

Yogurt dessert of your choice (page 288-304)

Day 18

Breakfast

Raw cocoa yogurt of your choice (page 298-301)

Grain: Natural organic oatmeal (page 271)

(or whole grain of your choice) (page 259)

Lunch

Salad: Very summery salad (page 235)

Main: Thai chicken soup (page 257)

Grain: Short grain coconut rice (page 260)

Yogurt Dessert

Matcha green tea yogurt of your choice (page 302-304)

Dinner

Soup/Complex starch: Red Lentil soup (page 246)

Main: Cod with stir-fried vegetables (page 205)

Dessert

Yogurt dessert of your choice (page 288-304)

Day 19

Breakfast

Matcha green tea yogurt of your choice (page 302-304)

Grain: Natural organic oatmeal (page 271)

(or whole grain of your choice) (page 259)

Lunch

Soup/Complex starch: Red lentil soup (page 246)

Main: Cod with stir-fried vegetables (page 205)

Yogurt Dessert

Cucumber watercress smoothie (page 295)

Dinner

Salad/Grain: Humus and crunchy vegetables (page 270)

Yogurt drink: Lassi (page 290)

Main: Tropical beef salad (page 225)

with mango chutney (page 278)

Breakfast

Raw cocoa yogurt of your choice (page 298-301)

Grain: Natural organic oatmeal (page 271)

(or whole grain of your choice) (page 259)

Lunch

Salad/Grain: Humus and crunchy vegetables (page 270)

Yogurt drink: Lassi (page 290)

Main: Tropical beef salad (page 225)

with mango chutney (page 278)

Dinner

Soup: Mom's cucumber yogurt soup (page 256)

Main: Asparagus with soft-cooked eggs (page 202)

Grain: Cilantro-lime rice (page 262)

Day 21

Breakfast

Matcha green tea yogurt of your choice (page 302-304)

Grain: Natural organic oatmeal (page 271)

(or whole grain of your choice) (page 259)

Lunch

Soup: Mom's cucumber yogurt soup (page 256)

Main: Asparagus with soft-cooked eggs (page 202)

Grain: Cilantro-lime rice (page 262)

Dinner

Salad: Coleslaw (page 242)

Main: Pork cutlets with caramelized onions and spinach (page 217)

Grain: saffron rice (page 266)

Yogurt Dessert

Cucumber watercress smoothie (page 288-304)

Day 22

Breakfast

Raw cocoa yogurt of your choice (page 298-301)

Grain: Natural organic oatmeal (page 271)

(or whole grain of your choice) (page 259)

Lunch

Salad: Coleslaw (page 242)

Main: Pork cutlets with caramelized onions and spinach (page 217)

Grain: Saffron rice (page 266)

Yogurt Dessert

Yogurt dessert of your choice (page 288-304)

Dinner

Vegetable/Complex starch: Stewed chickpeas

with tomato and zucchini (page 268)

Main: Curry chicken salad (page 207)

Yogurt Dessert

Yogurt dessert of your choice (288-304)

Day 23

Breakfast

Matcha green tea yogurt of your choice (page 302-304)

Grain: Natural organic oatmeal (page 271)

(or whole grain of your choice) (page 259)

Lunch

Vegetable/Complex starch: Stewed chickpeas

with tomato and zucchini (page 268)

Main: Curry chicken salad (page 207)

Yogurt Dessert

Yogurt dessert of your choice (page 288-304)

Dinner

Soup: Carrot soup (page 245)

Main/Complex starch: White bean salad with shrimp (page 200)

Yogurt Dessert

Yogurt and fruit (page 289)

Day 24

Breakfast

Raw cocoa yogurt of your choice (page 298-301)

Grain: Natural organic oatmeal (page 271)

(or whole grain of your choice) (page 259)

Lunch

Soup: Carrot soup (page 245)

Main/Complex starch: White bean salad with shrimp (page 200)

Yogurt Dessert

Yogurt and fruit (page 289)

Dinner

Salad: Maché and beet salad (page 229)

Main: Mexican chicken (page 224)

with guacamole (page 276)

Grain: Wild mix rice (page 259)

Yogurt Dessert

Yogurt dessert of your choice   (page 288-304)

Day 25

Breakfast

Matcha green tea yogurt of your choice (page 302-304)

Grain: Natural organic oatmeal (page 271)

(or whole grain of your choice) (page 259)

Lunch

Salad: Maché and beet salad (page 229)

Main: Mexican chicken (page 224)

with guacamole (page 276)

Grain: Wild mix rice (page 259)

Yogurt Dessert

Yogurt dessert of your choice   (page 288-304)

Dinner

Soup: Cream of zucchini   (page 247)

Main: Seared tuna with green beans (page 219)

Grain: Quinoa tabbouleh (page 267)

Day 26

Breakfast

Raw cocoa yogurt of your choice (page 298-301)

Grain: Natural organic oatmeal (page 271)

(or whole grain of your choice) (page 259)

Lunch

Soup: Cream of zucchini (page 247)

Main: Seared tuna with green beans (page 219)

Grain: Quinoa tabbouleh (page 267)

Dinner

Soup: Watercress cucumber summer soup (page 255)

Main: Indian tandoori chicken (page 222)

with spinach raita (page 239)

Grain: Jasmine rice (page 259)

Day 27

Breakfast

Matcha green tea yogurt of your choice (page 302-304)

Grain: Natural organic oatmeal (page 271)

(or whole grain of your choice) (page 259)

Lunch

Soup: Watercress cucumber summer soup (page 255)

Main: Indian tandoori chicken (page 222)

with spinach raita (page 239)

Grain: Jasmine rice (page 259)

Dinner (Vegetarian)

Soup/Complex starch: Minty green pea soup (page 254)

Main: Cucumber dill salad (page 237)

Grain: Millet couscous (page 265)

Yogurt Dessert

Yogurt dessert of your choice (page 288-304)

Day 28

Breakfast

Raw cocoa yogurt of your choice (page 298-301)

Grain: Natural organic oatmeal (page 271)

(or whole grain of your choice) (page 259)

Lunch (Vegetarian)

Soup/Complex starch: Minty green pea soup (page 254)

Main: Cucumber dill salad (page 237)

Grain: Millet couscous (page 265)

Yogurt Dessert

Yogurt dessert of your choice (page 288-304)

Dinner

Soup: Cream of asparagus (page 253)

Main: Fillet of beef with chimichurri (page 218)

and cherry tomato side salad

Grain: Red quinoa (page 259)

Day 29

Breakfast

Matcha green tea yogurt of your choice (page 302-304)

Grain: Natural organic oatmeal (page 271)

(or whole grain of your choice) (page 259)

Lunch

Soup: Cream of asparagus (page 253)

Main: Fillet of beef with chimichurri (page 218)

and cherry tomato side salad

Grain: Red quinoa (page 259)

Dinner

Soup/Complex starch: Braised lentils with eggplant (page 269)

Main: Toasted sesame seed chicken salad (page 209)

Yogurt Dessert

Yogurt dessert of your choice (page 288-304)

Day 30

Breakfast

Raw cocoa yogurt of your choice (page 298-301)

Grain: Natural organic oatmeal (page 271)

(or whole grain of your choice) (page 259)

Lunch

Vegetable/Complex starch: Braised lentils with eggplant (page 269)

Main: Toasted sesame seed chicken salad (page 209)

Yogurt Dessert

Yogurt dessert of your choice (page 288-304)

Dinner

Yougurt drink: Cucumber watercress smoothie (page 295)

Salad: New York salad (page 233)

Main: Oven roasted chicken with roasted vegetables (page 208)

Grain/Starch: Butternut squash

Breakfast

Matcha green tea yogurt of your choice (page 302-304)

Grain: Natural organic oatmeal (page 271)

(or whole grain of your choice) (page 259)

Lunch

Yogurt drink: Cucumber watercress smoothie (page 295)

Salad: New York salad (page 233)

Main: Oven roasted chicken with roasted vegetables (page 208)

Grain/Starch: Butternut squash

Dinner

Soup: Tortilla soup (page 251)

Yogurt drink: Lassi (page 290)

Main: Ceviche of monkfish (page 221)

with spicy mango chutney (page 278)

Grain: Coconut rice (page 260)

Day 32

Breakfast

Raw cocoa yogurt of your choice (page 298-301)

Grain: Natural organic oatmeal (page 271)

(or whole grain of your choice) (page 259)

Lunch

Soup: Tortilla soup (page 251)

Yogurt drink: Lassi (page 290)

Main: Ceviche of monkfish   (page 221)

with spicy mango chutney (page 278)

Grain: Coconut rice (page 260)

Dinner

Salad: Quick and light salad (page 234)

Main: Nutty chicken in creamy Indian spice (page 214)

with cucumber raita (page 238)

Grain/Starch: Brown basmati rice (page 259)

Day 33

Breakfast

Matcha green tea yogurt of your choice (page 302-304)

Grain: Natural organic oatmeal (page 271)

(or whole grain of your choice) (page 259)

Lunch

Salad: Quick and light salad (page 234)

Main: Nutty chicken in creamy Indian spice (page 214)

with cucumber raita (page 238)

Grain/Starch: Brown basmati rice (page 259)

Dinner

Soup: Cream of vegetable (page 252)

Main: Sea bass (page 198)

with dad's garlicky tomato salad (page 230)

Grain: Saffron rice (page 266)

Yogurt Dessert

Yogurt dessert of your choice (page 288-304)

Breakfast

Raw cocoa yogurt of your choice (page 298-301)

Grain: Natural organic oatmeal (page 271)

(or whole grain of your choice) (page 259)

Lunch

Soup: Cream of vegetable (page 252)

Main: Sea bass (page 198)

with dad's garlicky tomato salad (page 230)

Grain: Saffron rice (page 266)

Yogurt Dessert

Yogurt dessert of your choice (page 288-304)

Dinner

Yogurt drink: Lassi (page 290)

Salad: Fennel and orange salad (page 236)

Main: French rack of lamb (page 223)

and green beans with almonds (page 241)

Grain: Millet couscous (page 265)

Day 35

Breakfast

Matcha green tea yogurt of your choice (page 302-304)

Grain: Natural organic oatmeal (page 271)

(or whole grain of your choice) (page 259)

Lunch

Yogurt drink: Lassi (page 290)

Salad: Fennel and orange salad (page 236)

Main: Chicken breast with chimichurri sauce (page 280)

and sautéd spinach

Grain: Basmati and wild rice pilaf (page 263)

Dinner

Soup: Gazpacho (page 249)

Main: Pan fried fish with oven roasted vegetables of choice

Grain: Basmati and wild rice pilaf (page 263)

Yogurt Dessert

Yogurt dessert of your choice

MAIN DISHES

All recipes serve 4, unless spcecified otherwise

Super Chicken Salad with Red Quinoa

Ingredients

Two, 8-10-ounce chicken breasts, sliced into strips against the gain

Extra Virgin Olive Oil, enough to cover the bottom of the pan

1 large Spanish onion, sliced into bite sized wedges

1 cup thinly cut green or red cabbage

1 cup snow peas, peel off the string on the side

2 carrots, halved and cut lengthwise

1 1/2 tablespoons sesame seeds

1 tablespoon agave

Fresh grated orange zest, for extra flavor

Salt and pepper to taste

Directions

Heat a large sauté pan over medium heat; cover the bottom with olive oil and sauté onion for 5 minutes. Add the carrots and cabbage and sauté for about 6 minutes. Set aside on a serving platter. Add a little olive oil to the same pan and sauté the chicken pieces. When almost cooked add the snow peas and sauté together for 4 minutes. Raise temperature to high and return all the vegetables and sesame seeds to the pan. Heat for one quick minute.

In a serving platter mix all the ingredients together: the quinoa, the chicken vegetable mix, agave, orange zest and sea salt. Don't over mix. Serve hot or at room temperature.

Grain: Serve with red quinoa (page 259)

Sea bass with Mango Salad

Sea bass

Ingredients

Four, 4-5-ounce sea bass fillets
1/3 cup oat flour
1 egg beaten
1 cup macadamia nuts, crushed

Directions

Preheat oven at 350F. Pat dry the fish fillets. Crush the macadamia nuts into small pieces in a mortar or food processor and transfer to a flat plate. Beat the egg with two pinches of fine sea salt and 1 tablespoon water. Put the oat flour on a flat plate. Cover each fillet lightly with flour and wet both sides of the fillets with egg, finally cover well with the crushed macadamia nuts, pressing the fish on them. Place them on an oven tray, previously brushed with coconut oil. Bake for 15-20 minutes. Serve with the mango salad and a handful of coconut sticky brown rice on each plate.

Mango Salad

Ingredients

1 mango, pitted and diced
4 hearts of palm, thickly sliced (bottled)
2 tablespoons shredded coconut, fresh or dried*
1 tablespoon cilantro, chopped
1/2 teaspoon fresh ginger juice
1/2 tablespoon lime juice
1 1/2 tablespoons extra virgin olive oil
Fine sea salt and pepper to taste

Directions

To extract ginger juice, crush ginger in a garlic press. In a large bowl, whisk together the lime and ginger juices and olive oil. Add the mango, shredded coconut, cilantro and the hearts of palm. Mix and refrigerate.

Note: If choosing fresh coconut, use a wine opener to draw three holes at the base of the shell and drain the water; with a hammer, crack the coconut open and scoop out the meat. Grate it with a cheese grater over a plate.
Alternatively, you may use good quality packaged, dried grated coconut flesh.

Grain: serve with coconut rice (page 260)

White Bean Salad with Shrimp

Ingredients

2 lbs. shrimp, with the shell
2.5 cups small white beans, cooked
1 small onion, chopped
1 large red or orange pepper, seeded and cubed
2 vine ripe tomatoes, seeded, cubed
6 tablespoons extra virgin olive oil
4 sprigs fresh cilantro, finely chopped
3 tablespoons lemon juice
Salt and pepper to taste

Directions

In a large pot filled with boiling salted water, cook the shrimp for 5 minutes, or longer depending on the size of the shrimp. When the skins turn bright orange drain in a colander, cool off and peel. In a large bowl, toss together the cooked beans, onion, tomato, pepper and cilantro. Add olive oil, lemon juice, salt and pepper. Mix together and refrigerate until ready to use. Divide the bean salad among the plates and serve the shrimp on top.

Grain/Starch: Serve with small white beans (page 258)

Beef Stew

Ingredients

1-1.5 lbs beef stew meat cut into chunky strips about 1 1/2 inches

3 bones, to add flavor

Extra virgin olive oil

1 medium onion cut in thin wedges

2 cloves garlic, minced

3 large plump juicy tomatoes

2 medium carrots, peeled and cut lengthwise into 2 inch sticks

2 celery stalks, peeled and sliced crosswise

1 tablespoon red lentils, as a thickening agent

1/2 tablespoon fresh thyme (or 1 tablespoon dried)

1 bay leaf

1 tablespoon paprika

1 1/2 cups boiling water

Salt and black pepper to taste

Directions

Preheat the oven to 350°F. Place a casserole or Dutch oven on the stove at medium high heat, cover the bottom of the pot with olive oil, and sear the meat quickly in small batches, browning the meat on all sides. Remove the meat to a plate. Add the vegetables, bay leave and thyme to the pot. Cook for about 10 minutes, turning the vegetables. Add more olive oil as necessary and stir in the red lentils, return the meat to the casserole, pour the water over, add salt and pepper to taste. Cover with the lid and braise in the oven for 2.5 hours.

Grain/Starch: Serve with black lentils (page 258)

Asparagus with Soft-Cooked Eggs

Ingredients

1-2 medium eggs per person, soft-cooked
Extra virgin olive oil
16 thick asparagus, trimmed and bottoms peeled
Juice of 1 lemon
2 sprigs of each, rosemary and thyme, minced

Directions

Cooking perfect eggs every time has its little tricks. To achieve soft and runny yolks yet firm whites, follow these easy directions.

Place the eggs in one layer on the bottom of a saucepan. Cover with warm tap water going over one inch. Bring water to a rapid boil, cover the saucepan and remove form the heat. Let the eggs cook in the hot water for 3-4 minutes (depending on the size) for soft-cooked or up to 14 minutes for hard-cooked eggs.

Sauté the asparagus over medium heat for 8 minutes, shaking the pan frequently. Remove and serve on plates. Drizzle with lemon juice and olive oil. Peel the eggs and halve them lengthwise over the asparagus. Season with salt and pepper to taste and serve right away with a scoop of rice.

Grain: Serve with cilantro-lime (Recipe on page 262)

White Bean Stew with Scallops

Ingredients

1-1.5 lbs. large or small scallops

Extra virgin Olive oil

2 cups small white beans, cooked

6 cups filtered water

1 Spanish onion, peeled

1 ripe plum tomato

1 smallish carrot, peeled

3 sprigs fresh parsley

Salt and pepper to taste

Directions

Soak beans over night covered with water. The following day, drain and rinse under cool running water. In a large stockpot, combine the beans with the water and bring to a boil. Reduce heat to a simmer and add the onion, tomato, carrot, and parsley. Cook until tender, about 35 minutes. Be sure the beans are always covered with water. Add a little more water if the beans are getting too dry. When the beans are tender remove from the heat. Transfer the vegetables and 1/2 cup cooked beans to a food processor with 1/3 cup of its cooking liquid. Blend until creamy. Place a strainer over the stockpot containing the remaining beans and pass the vegetable mixture trough, pressing with the back of a spoon. Add two tablespoons of olive oil and season with sea salt. Bring back to a simmer. Just before ready to serve, sauté the scallops over medium heat with one tablespoon olive oil, about 3 minutes on each side, until golden brown. Place a ladleful of beans on individual plates and arrange the scallops on top. Drizzle a little olive oil and serve.

Albacore Tuna with Roasted Peppers and Garbanzo Bean Salad

Ingredients

Four, 4-5-ounce fresh white tuna steaks
2 red peppers, oven roasted
2 yellow peppers, oven roasted
8 garlic cloves, crushed and oven roasted
16 leaves of parsley
1/2 lemon juice
Sea salt and pepper, to taste

Directions

Preheat oven at 425° F. Place the whole peppers and garlic on an oven sheet, drizzle with olive oil and salt to taste. Roast for 30 minutes. Remove from the oven, transfer to a bowl and cool off. Peel, de-seed and cut the peppers into strips. Peel the garlic cloves and toss them into the bowl with the peppers. Drizzle generously with olive oil and lemon juice. Fold in the garbanzo beans. Set aside until ready to serve. Pat dry the tuna steaks and brush with olive oil. Bring a heavy-bottomed skillet to medium high heat and cook the tuna steaks 4 minutes on each side for medium rare. Place in a preheated oven for 20 minutes for well done.

Spoon the pepper and garbanzo salad over individual plates and place a fish steak on top. Garnish with a few leaves of parsley.

Grain/Starch: Serve with garbanzo beans (page 258)

Cod with Stir Fried Vegetables

Ingredients

Four, 4-5-ounce cod filets, or another white fish

Extra virgin olive oil

6 asparagus, trimmed and bottoms peeled

1 medium zucchini, cut into sticks

1/2 cup snow peas

1 small white onion, wedged

1 small red bell pepper, sliced lengthwise

1 red chili pepper (optional), sliced

2 tablespoons cilantro

Salt and pepper to taste

Directions

Preheat oven at 350°.   Bring a pan to medium high heat and cover the bottom with olive oil. Cook the cod fillets skin side down first, without over crowding the pan. After 7 minutes shake the pan, and when the steaks move freely, slide them over onto an oven sheet skin side up. Repeat as needed with the rest of the steaks and pour over any juices from the pan. Sprinkle with sea salt to taste. Transfer the tray to the oven and cook between 15 to 20 minutes. Meanwhile, in a sautéing pan, heat a little olive oil and cook each of the vegetables separately, adding more oil with each batch as needed. Be mindful not to over cook the vegetables, they must remain crispy. When the fish is done, place each steak on individual plates and serve with the vegetables.

Garnish with chopped cilantro and chili pepper

Pisto with Fried Eggs

Ingredients

2 eggs per person*
Extra virgin olive oil
4 garlic cloves, crushed with skin
1 Spanish onion, peeled and minced
1 green pepper, seeded and sliced lengthwise
2 medium zucchinis, diced
4 vine ripe tomatoes, diced
1 sprig fresh thyme
4 sprigs fresh parley, finely chopped
Salt and pepper to taste

Directions

Bring a sauté pan to medium heat and cover with abundant olive oil. Add the onions and thyme and cook until soft. Then add the garlic and sauté for 45 seconds. Toss in the pepper and cook for 2 minutes, then the zucchini until just soft. Incorporate the tomatoes and season to taste. Stew covered for 20 minutes. Spoon the pisto on individual plates and serve the eggs on top. Sprinkle with parsley.

To cook the eggs: Heat a sauté pan over medium heat and cover the bottom with abundant olive oil. It is very important that the pan is hot enough so that the eggs don't stick to the bottom. Break two eggs over the pan and cook until the edges of the whites are slightly crispy. Remove with a slotted flat spoon and serve over the pisto sauce. Repeat with the rest of the eggs. You may keep the plates in a warm oven until they are all ready to be served.

Note: Adults should eat 2 eggs. Substitute fried eggs for hard or soft-cooked eggs if you're making this dish in advance to take with you for lunch the next day (page 202.) Fried eggs taste best when cooked and eaten immediately.

Grain/Starch: Serve with sticky brown rice (page 259)

Curry Chicken Salad

Ingredients

1-1.5 lb. chicken breasts, diced
1/2 cup home-made mayonnaise (page 279)
1 teaspoon curry powder
4 celery stalks, peeled and finely chopped
1 tablespoon fresh cilantro, chopped
4 spring onions, white part only, thinly sliced
1 teaspoon coconut oil
1/2 teaspoon agave
2 Boston lettuces or another soft leaf lettuce
Sea salt and pepper to taste

Directions

Heat a pan over medium low heat and sauté the chicken pieces in olive oil until just golden on all sides. Set aside and cool off. Make mayonnaise plus add 1 teaspoon of curry powder and blend well. Combine the chicken, celery, green onions, cilantro and agave with the curry mayonnaise. Salt and pepper to taste.

Using the largest leaves of the lettuce, scoop equal parts of the chicken curry salad onto the centre and roll up tightly. As an alternative and less labor intensive, tear the leaves into bite size pieces, make a bed of lettuce onto each individual plate and scoop the chicken curry on top.

Oven Roasted Chicken

Ingredients

One 3 1/2-4 lb free-range whole chicken, giblets removed
1 lemon, halved
1 medium onion, peeled and whole
4 cloves garlic, unpeeled and crushed
2 sprigs rosemary
2 bay leaves
Salt and pepper
1 1/2 cups fresh (or frozen) green peas, shelled
4 carrots, cut into 1 inch pieces

Directions

Preheat oven at 425°F. Remove and discard excess fat from the chicken's bottom cavity. Rinse the chicken well under running cold water and pat dry with paper towels. Insert half the lemon inside the bird's back cavity, then the onion, garlic cloves, bay leaves, and the other half of the lemon at the end to keep it all in place. Place the chicken breast side up on a roasting pan and cover the skin with sea salt and fresh ground pepper.
Roast in the center rack.
Cut both ends of the squash, half lengthwise, discard the seeds, peel off the skin with a peeler and cut into wedges. Mix in with the rest of the vegetables in a bowl, drizzle with olive oil and season with salt. When the chicken begins to turn slightly golden, about 1 hour, toss the squash, carrots and green peas into the roasting pan. Continue cooking for another 30 minutes or until the skin on the chicken is crispy.
Transfer the chicken to a cutting board and let rest for 5 minutes.
Carve out the white meat and reserve the rest of the chicken to make soup or stock. Serve with the vegetables. Add salt and pepper to taste.

Note: I like to use the legs and carcass to make a delicious chicken soup or stock to eat the next day or freeze to have handy for when needed.

Toasted Chicken with Sesame Seeds

Ingredients

Two, 8-10-ounce chicken breasts, boneless, skinless

Extra virgin olive oil, for frying

1/2 cup oat flour

1 egg, beaten with one teaspoon water

1 cup sesame seeds

Assorted lettuces, such as Boston lettuce, red endive, yellow endive, frisé

Dressing:

2 tablespoons extra virgin olive oil

2 tablespoons sesame oil

1/2 teaspoon agave

2 tablespoons lemon juice

1/2 teaspoon mustard powder

1 teaspoon ginger juice

Grated zest of 1/2 lemon

Grated zest of 1/2 orange

Red pepper flakes

Salt to taste

Directions

In a large bowl whisk together the ingredients for the dressing and refriger-ate until ready to use. Cut the chicken breasts against the grain into 1/2-inch thick strips. Arrange four plates on a counter, one for the oat flour, one for the egg, another for the sesame seeds, and an empty one for the breaded chicken pieces. Season the egg and flour with salt and pepper, then cover the chicken lightly with each one of the ingredients on the plates. Heat a pan over medium heat and cover generously with olive oil. Fry the chicken until golden on both sides. Let stand on paper towels in a warm oven until the rest of the chicken is cooked. Cut the lettuces in thin strips and toss into the bowl with the dressing. Make a bed of lettuce on each plate and distribute a few pieces of chicken. Drizzle the rest of the dressing over.

Crab Salad

Ingredients

2 whole crabs, about 1.5 lbs each*
2 hard-coked eggs, peeled and finely chopped (Recipe on page XXX)
1cup grated coconut, loosely packed**
1 1/2 tablespoon ginger, peeled and grated
4 sprigs onions, discard green tops and slice
Zest of 2 limes, grated
1/2 tablespoon coconut oil
1 tablespoon extra virgin olive oil
4 cups chopped Boston lettuce, shredded

For the dressing:
4 tablespoons limejuice
8 tablespoons extra virgin olive oil
Salt and pepper to taste

Directions

Use a cheese grater to grate the coconut, ginger and lemon zest. Mix well.
In a sauté pan, over medium low heat, add the coconut and olive oils and cook the green onions until soft. Add the grated coconut mix and cook for 4 minutes, until aromatic. Set aside in a mixing bowl with the chopped eggs. Empty out the contents of the crab into the bow, helping with one of the crab's claws, and blend together with the coconut mix.
In a small bowl whisk the olive oil and lemon juice with salt to taste. Make a bed of lettuce on individual plates, divide the crab salad onto each plate and spoon over the dressing.

Note: Ask your fishmonger to clean the crab for you. He/she will give you the cracked legs and body with the meat, which you will have to empty out. You will need a total of 1 pound of crabmeat.

** If choosing fresh coconut-use a wine opener to draw three holes on the base of the shell and drain the water; crack the coconut open with a hammer and scoop out the meat. Grate it with a cheese grater over a plate. Alternatively, you may use organic, packaged, dried grated coconut.

Salmon with Roasted Sweet Pepper Sauce

Ingredients

1-1.5 lb. wild salmon, cut into fillets
Extra virgin olive oil, to cook the salmon
3 medium red bell peppers, roasted, seeded and peeled
1/3 cup extra-virgin olive oil, for the sauce
10 fresh basil leaves, shredded

Directions

Preheat the oven at 425°F. Brush the peppers with olive oil. Place them in a baking sheet and roast for 20-25 minutes. Take them out of the oven and set aside to cool off. Discard the tops, peel and deseed them. Place the peppers with its juices in a blender plus 1/3 cup olive oil and purée to a creamy sauce. Transfer to a small saucepan and season with salt and pepper to taste. Just before serving reheat at very low heat and stir in the basil.

Season the salmon with salt and pepper. Heat a sauté pan at medium high heat and cover the bottom generously with olive oil. Without overcrowding the pan, cook the salmon fillets on both sides until they easily slide off the pan when you shake it and the meat and skin are golden and crispy on the outside, yet pink inside. About 6 minutes on each side.

Spoon the sauce around each plate and place the salmon on top with a cup of black rice.

Grain/Starch: Serve with black rice if available, or a grain of your choice. (page 259)

Thai Tuna Carpaccio

Ingredients

1 pound sashimi-quality fresh tuna, very thinly sliced
1/2 cup extra virgin olive oil
1 teaspoon sesame seeds
16 drops Asian sesame oil
1/4 cup lime or lemon juice
1/4 teaspoon freshly ground black pepper
3 tablespoons fresh cilantro leaf, minced
1 tablespoon chives, very thinly sliced

Directions

Buy the freshest fish at the fish market. Don't sacrifice on quality. Cut
the tuna steaks against the grain into very thin slices. Whisk together the
olive oil, lemon juice and black pepper in a bowl. Pour half of the dressing
onto a large flat plate and arrange the tuna on top, then spoon the rest
of the dressing over the fish. Cover with plastic wrap and refrigerate for
20 minutes. Place the tuna pieces around individual plates with some of
the olive oil/lime marinade and drizzle a few drops of Asian sesame oil.
Sprinkle the sesame seeds, cilantro and chives. Serve cold.

Nutty Chicken in Indian Spices

Ingredients

1-1.5 lbs chicken breast cut in 1-inch cubes
Extra virgin olive oil
4 garlic cloves, finely chopped
1 medium onion
1/2 cup raw almonds
1/3 cup raw pistachios, shelled
1 inch piece ginger, finely chopped
1/3 cup water or chicken stock
1 large pinch saffron threads
1/2 teaspoon cinnamon
1/2 teaspoon cardamom
1/2 teaspoon cumin
Salt and pepper to taste
2/3 cup plain yogurt

Directions

Chop the almonds and pistachios finely in a food processor or blender. Be careful not to turn them into a paste. Dissolve the saffron in a little bit of water. Heat a pan over medium low heat and sauté the onion in olive oil until golden. Add the garlic, ginger and chicken. Cook for 5 minutes stirring constantly, then add the spices with the saffron and mix well. Pour over the water or chicken stock and season with salt and pepper to taste. Cover and simmer for 20 minutes. Uncover and toss in the crushed nuts and continue cooking covered for another 10 minutes. Simmer uncovered for 10 more minutes. Remove from the heat and let rest for 12 minutes before folding in the yogurt.
Serve over jasmine rice and a refreshing mint cucumber raita
on the side (page 238).

Grain: Serve with brown jasmine rice (page 259)

Peruvian Style Chicken

Ingredients

1-1.5 lbs. chicken breast, cubed
Extra virgin olive oil
4 tablespoons extra virgin olive oil, for the chili pepper oil
1 red or orange chili pepper, seeded and sliced, optional
1 red onion, chopped
1 1/2 tablespoons garlic, minced
1/3 teaspoon cumin
1/2 cup water
1/2 cup limejuice, fresh squeezed
1/2 cup oat flour
1/2 cup almonds, ground
3 cups chicken stock or filtered water
2 tablespoons olive oil
Salt and pepper to taste

Directions

To make pepper oil blend together 4 tablespoons olive oil with the sliced chili pepper in a mortar or food processor. In a bowl, mix the chicken pieces with 1 tablespoon crushed garlic, 2 tablespoons pepper oil and cumin, then season with salt and pepper. Pour over the limejuice and 1/2 cup water. Marinate for 30 minutes in the refrigerator. In a sauté pan over medium heat, cover the bottom with olive oil and sauté the onion until translucent. Add the remaining tablespoon garlic and sauté for 45 seconds, until the ingredients are just turning golden. Add the rest of the pepper oil and cook for another 2 minutes. Pour the water or chicken stock and bring the sauce back to a boil, reduce the heat and simmer gently. Drain the chicken and pat dry, then coat lightly with oat flour. In a separate pan over medium heat, cover the bottom with olive oil and sauté the chicken until cooked through and golden, about 10 minutes. Transfer the chicken to the saucepan, add the almonds and blend together. Serve warm, over rice.

Grain/Starch: Serve with basmati brown rice (page 259)

Minced Meat with Tomatoes and Eggplant

Ingredients

1-1.5 lb minced meat
Extra virgin olive oil
1 large yellow onion, wedged
3 garlic cloves, crushed with the skin on
3 medium tomatoes on the vine, wedged
3 cups eggplant, thinly sliced
1 teaspoon Spanish sweet paprika
1/2 teaspoon mustard powder
2 tablespoons pine nuts
5 fresh thyme sprigs, leaves only
Salt and pepper to taste

Directions

Heat a pan at medium low heat and cover the bottom with a generous amount of olive oil. Sauté the onions until tender, then add the garlic and sauté for 45 seconds. Stir in the tomatoes and cook until tender. Place the eggplant slices around the pan and mix the rest of the ingredients together, sending the eggplant to the bottom. Keep a watchful eye on the vegetables and stir frequently. Break down the vegetables with the edge of the spatula to turn them into a mush. Add the mustard and paprika, and cook at low heat uncovered in its juices for about 10 more minutes. Transfer to a bowl and set aside.

Bring the pan back to medium high heat, cover the bottom lightly with olive oil and sauté the minced meat until lightly browned. About 6 minutes. Mix in the meat with the vegetables in the bowl and serve over rice on individual plates sprinkled with the thyme and pine nuts.

Grain: Serve with wild rice mix (page 259)

Pork Cutlets with Caramelized Onions

Ingredients

1-1.5 lbs. natural boneless pork loin
Extra virgin olive oil
2 Spanish onions, sliced
4 handfuls loose spinach leaves
Salt and pepper to taste

Directions

Tell your butcher to trim off the fat of the loin. Pat dry with paper towels, cut into medallions, 2 to 3-ounces each. Brush with olive oil and season with salt and pepper.

Heat a heavy bottom skillet over medium low heat. Drizzle olive oil over the onions and salt them lightly. Cook the onions until golden on both sides and caramelized. Set aside on a platter in a warm oven. Return the heavy bottom skillet to medium high heat and sear the pork cutlets, about 6 minutes on each side. If you're cooking the medallions in batches, keep them warm in the oven at low temperature with the onions. On a clean pan, sauté the spinach quickly with a little olive oil, about 3 minutes. Serve a handful of the onions on each plate and place 2-3 medallions on top. Serve with spinach and saffron rice on the side.

Note: Pork tastes best when it's a little pink inside. But if you like it cooked all the way through, then set the oven at 450° and finish cooking the meat in the oven for 15 minutes.

Grain: Serve with saffron rice (page 266)

Fillet Mignon with Chimichurri Sauce

Ingredients

4 beef filets, 4-5 ounce each
8 garlic cloves, crushed and with the skin on
5 ounces baby spinach

Chimichurri Sauce:
1 cup fresh Italian parsley leaves, minced
1/2 cup olive oil
1/3 cup lemon juice
1/2 lemon rind, grated
1/4 cup fresh cilantro leaves, minced
2 garlic cloves, peeled
3/4 teaspoon dried crushed red pepper
1/2 teaspoon ground cumin
1/2 teaspoon salt

Directions

Preheat oven at 450°. Heat an ovenproof heavy skillet over medium high heat. When the skillet is smoky hot place the fillets and sear for 3 minutes on each side. Transfer the skillet with the meat to the oven and cook for 10 minutes for medium rare and 16 minutes for medium.
Sauté the spinach on a medium heated pan with olive oil, about 3 minutes. Serve the meat right away on individual plates, seasoned with salt and plenty of fresh pepper. Spoon over some chimichurri sauce and serve with the spinach and quinoa.

Chimichurri Sauce
Whisk all the ingredients together in a bowl until well mixed. Serve at room temperature. You can prepare this sauce ahead of time.

Grain: Serve with red quinoa (page 259)

Seared Tuna with Green Beans and Almonds

Ingredients

1-1.5 lbs albacore tuna steaks, 2 or 4 steaks
2 teaspoons extra virgin olive oil
4 scallions, finely slivered
1/2 cup cilantro leaves, minced
1/2 cup mint leaves, minced
4 lime wedges
Sea salt and pepper
Green beans (page 241)

Dressing:
2 teaspoons extra virgin olive oil
10 drops Asian sesame oil
2 teaspoons lemon juice
1 teaspoon grated ginger
1/3 cup cilantro leaves
Salt and pepper to taste

Directions

In a food processor blend together all the ingredients for the dressing. Brush the tuna steaks with olive oil and season with salt and pepper to taste. Heat a heavy skillet over medium heat. When the pan is hot, add the steaks and cook for 5 minutes on each side. Serve with green beans. Sprinkle with scallions, cilantroand mint, then pour over the dressing. Serve with a lemon wedge on the side.

Note: If you prefer the tuna well-done, bake in a 450° oven for an extra 15 minutes.

Grain: Serve with cilantro- lime basmati rice (page 262)

Chicken Stir-Fry with Red Pepper Broccoli and Bock Choy

Ingredients

1-1.5 lbs. skinless chicken breast, thinly sliced against the grain

1 teaspoon extra virgin olive oil

2 teaspoons cold pressed sesame oil

8 medium broccoli florets

1 tablespoon freshly grated ginger

1/2 clove garlic, crushed

1 medium onion, quartered

1 red bell pepper, seeded and sliced

1 head broccoli florets, separated

2 bunches baby bock choy, discard toughest white part

2 teaspoons sesame seeds

Directions

Bring a sauté pan to medium heat and cover the bottom lightly with olive and sesame oils. Sauté the garlic and ginger for 20 seconds and add the chicken to stir-fry for 8 minutes, until golden. Set aside. Add more olive and sesame oils to the pan and sauté the onion and red pepper for 5 minutes. Set aside. Add bock choy and broccoli and sauté until tender. Return all the ingredients to the pan with the sesame seeds, and reheat stirring constantly for 2 minutes.

Serve with sticky brown rice (page 259)

Ceviche of Monkfish

Ingredients

1 lb. monkfish fillets; you may use another white fish
3 tablespoons extra virgin olive oil
 Juice of 4 limes
1 medium red hot chili pepper, halved and seeded
1 small red onion, sliced paper thin
2 tablespoons cilantro, minced
Sea salt to taste
Serve with guacamole (page 276) or mango chutney (page 278)

Directions

Cut the fish fillets against the grain into thin slices, place them in a shallow glass container with the onions and cover well with the limejuice, adding more juice if needed. Cover with plastic wrap and refrigerate for 20-30 minutes. Just before serving, lift the fish carefully with a slotted spoon from of the limejuice and gently toss together with the chili and cilantro. Divide the ceviche into four portions and scoop onto each plate. Serve right away with guacamole on the side.

Note: The lime juice where the fish has been marinated can be served chilled on a shot glass on the side. This is considered a medicinal elixir in South and Central America.

Tandoori Chicken with Spinach Raita

Ingredients

1.25 lb. boneless skinless chicken breast, cut into 1-inch cubes
Extra virgin olive oil
1 1/2 tablespoons curry powder
1 tablespoon lemon juice
1 tablespoon Spanish paprika
1/2 teaspoon ground cumin
2 large cloves garlic, peeled
1inch ginger, peeled
1 medium Spanish onion, minced
1 1/4 cup yogurt
1/2 cup cilantro leaves, minced
Salt to taste
Lemon wedges, for garnish
8 bamboo skewers, soaked in warm water for 30 minutes
Serve with spinach raita (page 239)

Directions

In a food processor, mix together the curry powder, lemon juice, paprika, cumin, garlic, ginger, onion and yogurt. Transfer to a glass container, toss in the chicken pieces and coat well. Refrigerate between 2 and 3 hours.
Preheat oven to 350°F. Drain the chicken and thread the pieces into the skewers. Reserve the marinade. Cover the bottom of a pan over high heat with olive oil and sear the chicken until golden, about 1 minute on each side. Transfer to a baking sheet and bake for 10 minutes. Meanwhile, bring the marinade to a slow boil in a saucepan. Place the chicken skewers on individual plates, spoon over the yogurt sauce and sprinkle with cilantro. Serve with rice and cucumber raita.

Grain: Serve with jasmine brown rice (page 259)

French Rack of Lamb

Ingredients

Two, 1 lb French cut racks of lamb, 3 to 4 ribs per person
1/4 cup extra virgin olive oil
2 large garlic cloves, minced
1/2 tablespoon crushed mixed pepper seeds
2 tablespoons fresh rosemary, finely chopped
Green beans with almonds (page 241)
Sea salt to taste

Directions

Ask your butcher to trim off any excess fat and leave just a thin layer.
Preheat oven at 375°F. In a small bowl, mix together the olive oil, garlic, rosemary and pepper, rub the mixture over the side of the lamb with the fat, pressing with the back of a spoon to adhere the mixture well to the surface. Heat an ovenproof skillet over medium heat until you see smoke. Sear the lamb, fat side down, first, turn it over and cook for about 3 minutes on each side. Transfer to the oven and roast between 15-20 minutes for medium rare*. Transfer to a cutting board and let it sit for 4 minutes. Then cut each rib and serve with green beans and couscous on the side.

*Note: Lamb should be eaten pink inside. Not only is it tastier and juicer, it actually also holds more nutrients and enzymes.

Grain: Serve with millet couscous (page 265)

Mexican chicken

Ingredients

1.25 lb. chicken breasts, sliced against the grain into strips
Extra virgin olive oil
1/2 cup lime juice
4 garlic cloves, bruised
1/2 teaspoon chili powder
1 teaspoon dried oregano
1/2 teaspoon dried thyme
1 red pepper, seeded and cut into strips
1 green pepper, seeded and cut into strips
2 medium onions, thinly sliced
1/2 cup Greek yogurt
Salt and fresh pepper to taste
Guacamole (page 276)

Directions

Mix together the limejuice, herbs, garlic, salt and pepper. Add the chicken pieces and marinate for 3 hours (or up to 12 hours) in the refrigerator. Remove the chicken with a slotted spoon and place on a dish with paper towels. Mix the vegetables in the same marinade. Bring a heavy skillet over medium high heat, drizzle the bottom with olive oil and cook the chicken, in batches if necessary, not to overcrowd the pan, about 10 minutes. Set aside on a plate. Take the vegetables out of the marinade with a slotted spoon (discard the marinade) and add to the hot pan with a drizzle of olive oil. Cook for 8 minutes stirring frequently. Toss the chicken back into the pan and sauté for 1 minute. Serve right away with basmati rice and guacamole. Scoop some of the yogurt on the side as a substitute for sour cream.

Grain: Serve with basmati rice (page 259)

Tropical Beef Salad

Ingredients

Two, 8 Oz New York steaks, naturally raised
4 lose cups arugula leaves
1 red pepper, seeded and finely sliced
4 scallions, finely sliced
1/3 cup cilantro leaves
2 tablespoons chopped mint
Mango chutney (page 278)

Marinade
2 tablespoons extra virgin olive oil
1 tablespoon agave nectar
1 teaspoon ginger juice
1/3 teaspoon cumin
1 large clove garlic, minced
1 1/2 teaspoons fresh milled pepper
Salt to taste

Dressing
1 1/2 tablespoons extra virgin olive oil
1 1/2 teaspoons lime juice
1 red chili pepper, and sliced thinly
Salt and pepper to taste

Directions

To make the marinade, whisk together the olive oil, agave, ginger juice, cumin, garlic, salt and pepper in a bowl. Spread the mixture on a large flat plate and coat the steaks well on both sides.

Heat a heavy-bottom pan on medium high heat until hot. Place the steaks and cook for 5 minutes on each side for rare, or 7 minutes for medium rare. Reserve the juices. Set aside for 8 minutes. Transfer to a cutting board, discard any large fat around the edges and slice the steaks thinly against the grain.

In a large bowl mix the olive oil, lime juice and chili pepper. Toss in the arugula, red pepper, scallions, cilantro and mint. Serve on individual salad plates with the meat slices folded on top. Spoon over the meat juices. Season with salt and pepper and serve with mango chutney on the side.

SALADS

If you're planning on eating the salad later or the next day, reserve the dressing and pour it over the salad at the moment you're ready to eat it. Otherwise you will end up with a very oily and soggy salad. You want the salad to be fresh and crisp

Tomato Cucumber Kefir Salad

Ingredients

Serves 4

1 1/2 cups kefir*
2 large green onions, minced
2 Persian cucumbers, seeded and diced
2 medium salad tomatoes, seeded and diced
1 1/2 tablespoons cilantro leaves, minced
1 1/2 tablespoons olive oil
1 tablespoon lime juice
Salt and pepper to taste

Directions

In a medium size bowl blend together the kefir, olive oil, lime juice, salt and pepper. Fold in the onions, cucumbers and tomatoes. Sprinkle with cilantro.

*Note: Alternatively you may use yogurt.

Caesar Salad

Ingredients

1 large romaine lettuce, with very green leaves
2 large garlic cloves, minced
6 tablespoons olive oil
2 organic egg yolks, at room temperature
1 teaspoon mustard powder
Juice of 1 lemon
Sea salt to taste
Freshly milled black pepper

Directions

Buy a plush and thick romaine lettuce. Wash the lettuce leaves well, pat dry and refrigerate. Submerge the eggs carefully in boiling water for 45 seconds. Crack open and separate the yolks from the whites, discarding the later. In a large bowl, whisk together the egg yolks, garlic, lemon juice, mustard powder and sea salt. Place 4 or 5 large lettuce leaves on individual plates and spoon the dressing over.
Serve immediately with pepper.

Note: Scared of salmonella? Salmonella is found in the eggshell, nothing boiling water can't kill. Lemon also kills salmonella. Interesting to note that recipes that call for raw eggs, such as mayonnaise also call for lemon. A coincidence? I would dare to say that it's a safety measure our ancestors left for us.

Maché and Beet Salad

Ingredients

4 medium size beets of assorted colors, roasted, peeled and quartered*
3 fresh thyme sprigs
1 1/2 tablespoons olive oil
4 bunches maché leaves, or another lose salad green
1 cup yogurt cheese balls (page 286)
3 tablespoons raw pistachios, shelled
Sea salt and fresh pepper

Dressing:
1/2 teaspoon mustard powder
3 tablespoons lemon juice
Zest of 1 orange
4 spring onions, thinly sliced
1/3 cup extra virgin olive oil
Salt and pepper

Directions

Preheat oven to 425°F. Brush the beets with olive oil, and place them on an oven pan with the garlic and thyme. Sprinkle about 2 tablespoons water over, season with salt and pepper and roast for 25 minutes. Let them cool off to room temperature.

For the dressing, whisk together the mustard, lemon juice, olive oil, orange zest, salt and pepper in a medium size bowl. Add the spring onions.

Peel off the beets, cut them in quarters and toss them into the bowl with the dressing until ready to eat. Keep refrigerated.

Make a bed with a handful of the green leaves on each plate, toss in the beets and the dressing. Arrange the yogurt cheese balls around the plates and sprinkle with pistachios or other raw nuts of your choice.

Note: For the raw beet salad alternative simply peel the beets and slice thinly.

Dad's Garlicky Tomato Salad

Ingredients

2 large heirloom salad tomatoes, cored and wedged
2 medium garlic cloves, minced
Extra virgin olive oil
Salt to taste

Directions

In a bowl mix the tomatoes and garlic, then drizzle with plenty of olive oil and salt to taste. Serve right away at room temperature.

Note: The secret to this easy to make salad is finding super flavorful firm, yet juicy tomatoes. The trick is to smell them and let your nose capture the beautiful earthy smell of a tomato. If it doesn't wrap you all around with its aroma, move on to the next batch. For this salad, there's not such a thing as too much garlic.

Mango Salad

Ingredients

1 large mango, pitted and diced

4 hearts of palm, sliced (bottled without preservatives added)

1 cup shredded coconut, preferably fresh

1 tablespoon cilantro, chopped

1/2 teaspoon fresh ginger juice

1/2 tablespoon lime juice

1 1/2 tablespoons extra virgin olive oil

Salt and pepper to taste

Directions

To extract ginger juice, peel and crush using a garlic press. In a large bowl, whisk together the lime and ginger juices and olive oil. Add the mango, shredded coconut, cilantro and hearts of palm. Serve as a side dish.

Green Bean Salad

Ingredients

1 pound green beans, steamed (haricots verts when available)

1 medium onion, minced

1 cup cherry tomatoes, halved

8 hard-cooked eggs, peeled and wedged (on page 202)

Juice of 2 lemons

6 tablespoons extra virgin olive

Salt and pepper

Directions

Steam the green beans for about 8 minutes total, depending on the thickness of the beans. In a bowl whisk together the olive oil, lemon, salt and pepper. Mix in the onions, tomatoes and green beans. Serve the salad on individual plates, pour over the dressing mix and divide the egg wedges among each plate.

New York Salad

Ingredients

2 green crispy apples, peeled and quartered

5 celery stalks, peeled and thinly sliced

2/3 cups raw walnut halves

Juice of 1/2 lemon

1 lemon zest

1 shallot, minced

1 small garlic clove, minced

5 large green romaine lettuce leaves, thinly sliced

2 handfuls frisé lettuce leaves, chopped

Dressing:

1 tablespoon lemon juice

1 teaspoon mustard powder

5 tablespoons olive oil

4 tablespoons Greek yogurt

Directions

Grate the zest of the lemon into a large bowl and squeeze all but 1 table-spoon of the juice. Mix in the apples, celery, shallot and garlic with the lemon juice. Refrigerate.

Dressing:

Place 1 tablespoon lemon juice in a small bowl and mix with the mustard. Whisk in the olive oil, a few drops at a time until smooth, then incorporate the yogurt and blend well together. Season with salt and pepper to taste.
Add the lettuce leaves to the apple salad and mix well. Serve right away with walnuts tossed on top.

Quick and Light Salad

Ingredients

1 head Boston lettuce, sliced
2 carrots, shredded
2 Persian cucumbers, shredded
1/2 cup cherry tomatoes, halved
1 large bunch pea sprouts, or another type
4 tablespoons pumpkin seeds
6 tablespoons olive oil
Juice of 1 lemon or lime
Salt and pepper

Directions

In a bowl, whisk together the olive oil, lemon juice, spring onions salt and pepper. Add the vegetables and mix well. Serve right away.

Note: This salad can have as many variations as you would like. Add avocados, green onions, nuts, yogurt cheese, etc.

Very Summery Salad

Ingredients

1 head yellow Belgian endive, cored and cut lengthwise into strips
1 head red Belgian endive, cored and cut lengthwise into strips
1 bunch fresh watercress, remove stems
1/4 cup walnut pieces*
1 cup yogurt cheese balls with fresh herbs of your choice

Vinaigrette:
3 tablespoons olive oil
Juice of 1/2 lemon
1/2 shallot, minced
1/2 teaspoon agave
Salt and pepper

Directions

Whisking together the olive oil, lemon juice and shallot in a large bowl, then season with salt and pepper to taste. Combine the vegetables in the bowl with the dressing. Serve the salad among individual plates with cheese balls and sprinkle with walnuts.

Note: : For deeper flavor, toast the walnuts on a pan over medium heat for 6 minutes.

Shaved Fennel and Orange Salad

Ingredients

4 handfuls frisé lettuce,
1 large fennel bulb
4 tablespoons pine nuts
1 blood orange or Valencia orange, peeled and wedged*

Dressing:
6 tablespoons extra virgin olive oil
3 tablespoons lemon juice
1 small shallot, minced
1/2 teaspoon rosemary, minced
Salt and pepper

Directions

In a big bowl, whisk the olive oil, lemon juice, rosemary and shallots. Set aside. Peel the orange and discard the thin skin layer that covers the wedges. Discard the stem of the fennel and keep only the most tender parts. Cut the bulb in halve lengthwise and cut crosswise into paper-thin slices. Toss in the frisé lettuce and fennel together with the dressing. Divide the salad among individual plates and add the orange wedges. Sprinkle with pine nuts.

Note: This salad is also delicious with grapefruit.

Cucumber Dill Salad

Ingredients

4 Persian cucumbers, thinly sliced*
1 clove garlic, minced
1/3 cup yogurt
1 tablespoon fresh lemon juice
3 tablespoons olive oil
2 tablespoons finely chopped fresh dill
Salt and pepper

Note: IIf you are using another type of cucumbers, peel and slice them.
You may substitute the dill for fresh mint to compliment better certain flavors.

Directions

In a bowl, whisk the yogurt, dill, garlic, lemon juice, salt and pepper. Add the olive oil and continue whisking until well blended. Toss in the cucumber and mix well. You may refrigerate for one hour before serving.

Cucumber raita

Ingredients

Serves 2
1cup plain yogurt
Extra virgin olive oil
3 Persian cucumbers, diced
1/8 teaspoon cumin powder
One large pinch of paprika, preferably the Spanish kind
2 teaspoons cilantro leaves, minced
Salt and pepper to taste

Directions

Whisk the yogurt. Add the cucumber, cumin, salt and pepper. Mix well. Drizzle a few drops of olive oil and serve cool, garnished with paprika and cilantro leaves.

A classical Indian side dish, raitas are a favorite of mine because they go well with pretty much any main dish. They're also very cooling and digestive, so it makes sense that in India, raita is served along side spicy foods. Traditionally they're made with yogurt, but I sometimes make them with kefir.

Spinach raita

Ingredients

Serves 2
1cup yogurt
A handful of spinach leaves, cut into strips
1/8 teaspoon cumin powder
One large pinch of paprika, preferably Spanish
Grated zest of 1/2 lemon
Salt and pepper to taste

Directions

Wash the spinach, drain and place in a hot pan and cook until wilted and deep green in color, about 3 minutes. Cool off in the refrigerator.
Whisk the yogurt with the cumin, paprika, lemon zest, salt and pepper in a medium bowl. Add the spinach and serve cool.

Tomato raita

Ingredients

Serves 2
1 cup plain yogurt
1 large tomato, seeded and cubed
1/8 teaspoon cumin powder
1 tablespoon onion, finely chopped
2 teaspoons cilantro leaves, minced
Salt and pepper to taste

Directions

Whisk the yogurt with cumin, salt and pepper. Mix in the tomato and onion. Serve cool, garnished with cilantro leaves.

Green Beans with Almonds

Ingredients

4 handful of green beans, trimmed (preferably haricots verts)
Extra virgin olive oil
1/2 cup slivered almonds
4 shallots thinly sliced
1/2 tablespoon fresh thyme.
Salt and pepper to taste

Directions

My favorite beans are the French variety haricots verts, because they're the most tender. If you can't find them, go with the regular kind, but be aware that they take a bit longer to cook.

Steam the beans until just tender, about 8 minutes, and set them aside. In a large frying pan over medium heat, toast the almonds, shaking constantly until golden brown. Set aside. Add olive oil to the pan and sauté the shallots until they begin to brown. At this point, stir in the beans and shake the pan for 2 minutes. Transfer to a plate, season with salt and pepper and toss in the almonds and thyme.

Coleslaw

Ingredients

1/2 head green cabbage, shredded

6 spring onions, white and light green part only, sliced

3 carrots, shredded

3 celery stalks, peeled and thinly sliced

Dressing:

1/3 cup mayonnaise (follow recipe on page XXX)

3 tablespoons Greek style yogurt

3 tablespoons extra virgin olive oil

1 tablespoon lemon

1/2 teaspoon dried mustard

1 clove garlic. Minced

1/2 teaspoon agave

Salt and pepper to taste

Directions

Combine mayonnaise with the yogurt, olive oil, lemon, mustard, garlic and agave and mix together. Add the cabbage, green onions, carrots and celery, and coat ingredients well with the dressing. Season to taste. Keep refrigerated until ready to use.

Note: This is a delicious salad that keeps well from one day to the next with the dressing added.

Greek Salad

Ingredients

3 vine ripe tomatoes, cut into wedges

1/3 red onion, thinly sliced

2 Persian cucumbers, cubed

1 green pepper, seeded and sliced

1 tablespoon parsley

1/2 cups herbed yogurt cheese

Dressing:

3 tablespoons extra virgin olive oil

1 1/2 tablespoons lemon juice

1 small clove garlic, minced

1/2 teaspoon dried oregano

Salt and pepper to taste

Directions

In a large bowl whisk together all the ingredients for the dressing. Add the vegetables and mix well. Serve on individual salad plates with yogurt cheese balls on top.

SOUPS

People are some times intimidated when faced with the task of making a soup. This is rather the easies of all dishes to make in the kitchen. And once you get the hang of it, you will quickly realize that you can come up with your own great soups without following a recipe.

Carrot Soup

Ingredients

Serves 4

3 tablespoons extra virgin olive oil

5 cups water, filtered

1 leek

1 large celery stalk

2 fresh parsley sprigs

1 fresh thyme sprig (or 1/2 tsp dried)

6 medium carrots, diced

1 teaspoon peppercorns

1/2 cup fresh cilantro

1/2 teaspoon turmeric

Salt to taste

Directions

Heat a medium size saucepan over medium-low heat; add olive oil, onion and garlic, reduce the heat to very low, and stir occasionally until tender and transparent in color, about 10 minutes. Cover with water and add the white portion of the leek and celery. Secure the bay leave, parsley and thyme sprigs inside the green leaves of the leek and add to the saucepan. Bring to medium-low heat and simmer for 15 minutes. Add the carrots and season with salt and pepper to taste. Simmer until carrots are tender, about 15 minutes. Allow to cool off. Discard the green part of the leek, herbs and celery. Purée the soup in small batches in a food processor or blender, and transfer back to the saucepan. Keep covered at a simmer heat until ready to serve. Sprinkle with fresh cilantro.

Red Lentil Soup

Serves 4

1 cup red lentils

4 tablespoons extra virgin olive oil

1 medium leek, white and light part only, thinly sliced

1 medium carrot, cubed

1 vine ripe tomato, cubed

1 bay leave

6 cups water, filtered

1 tablespoon cilantro leaves, chopped

3 key limes

Smoked sea salt (Matiz)

Fresh milled pepper

Directions

Rinse the red lentils under cold running water and drain. Heat the olive oil in a medium saucepan. Add the leek and cook at medium low heat until soft, about 8 minutes. Add the carrot, tomato and bay leaf and cook for 10 minutes until tender, stirring frequently. Pour in the lentils and mix well. Pour in the water, add the smoked salt and pepper and cook until the lentils are tender, about 35 minutes. Serve on soup plates with cilantro leaves and lime wedges.

Cream of Zucchini Soup

Ingredients

Extra virgin olive oil
4 medium zucchinis, cubed
1 medium onion, finely chopped
4 whole garlic cloves, minced
4 cups water, filtered
2 1/3 cups yogurt
Mint leaves, minced
Salt and pepper to taste

Directions

Heat a medium saucepan over medium low heat and cover the bottom with a generous amount of olive oil. Cook the onion until soft, then sauté the garlic for 45 seconds, until barely golden. Add the zucchini and cook slowly until tender, 15 minutes. Blend the mixture in batches in an electric mixer. Add a little water if necessary. Return to the pot and add the rest of the water to achieve a smooth creamy texture. Simmer for 10 minutes and then transfer to a glass bowl to cool off, about 20 minutes. Whisk in the yogurt an serve with mint leaves.

Eggplant Soup with Yogurt

Ingredients

Extra-virgin olive oil

1 large eggplant, peeled and cubed

1 large leek, white and light green part only, sliced

6 cups water, filtered

1 teaspoon smoked Spanish salt-Matiz

1 teaspoon cumin

1 tablespoon dill

1 tablespoon chives

1cup natural yogurt, Greek style

Salt and pepper to taste

Direction:

Over medium low heat, cover the bottom of a saucepan with olive oil. Cook the leek for about 7 minutes, stirring frequently. Toss in the eggplant in batches and cover well with olive oil, add more if necessary. Sprinkle the smoked salt and cumin and cook for 5 minutes. Pour in the water and simmer covered for 20 minutes. Blend in small batches in a blender or food processor until smooth and creamy. Serve warm (not too hot) with a dollop of cool Greek yogurt on top, sprinkled with dill and chives.

Gazpacho

Ingredients

1/4 cup olive oil
3 ripe beefsteak tomatoes
1/2 sweet red pepper
1 cucumber, peeled and seeded
1 large garlic clove
1/2 small onion
3 tablespoons olive oil
1/2 teaspoon Spanish sweet paprika
4 cups water, purified
Salt and pepper taste

For garnish:
1 lime, wedged
1 small Persian cucumber cut into very thin rounds
2 radishes, very thinly sliced
4 parsley sprigs

Directions

Blend together the tomatoes, red pepper, cucumber, garlic, onion, paprika, olive oil and salt with water in an electric mixer. If the consistency is too thick, add a little more water until the desired texture is achieved. Serve chilled in individual bowls, garnished with a few slices of cucumber and radishes, and a lemon wedge on the side to splash in the gazpacho if desired. Season with pepper.

Tip: To avoid garlic or onion breath, eat a small parsley sprig afterwards.

Butternut Squash Soup

Ingredients

Extra virgin olive oil

3/4 lb butternut squash, peeled, seeded and cubed

1/2 Spanish onion, minced

1/2 inch fresh ginger, grated

1 large tomato

Lemon peal of 1/2 lemon

1 pinch nutmeg

2 cups water

4 cups chicken stock

5 saffron threads mixed with 1tablespoon chicken stock (optional)

1 tablespoon cilantro, minced

Salt and pepper to taste

Directions

In a medium stockpot, heat oil over medium low heat, sauté onion until soft, about 10 minutes. Add ginger and cook for 2 minutes, then sauté the tomatoes for 8 minutes. Stir in the squash cubes with the rest of the ingredients, season with salt, pepper and nutmeg. Pour the chicken stock and water, and add the lemon peel. If using saffron, add it now, as well. Bring to a quick boil; reduce to a simmer and cover. Cook until the squash is tender, about 25 minutes. Let it cool off and blend in batches in an electric mixer until smooth and silky. Return to the stockpot and keep warm. Garnish with cilantro.

Tortilla Soup

Extra virgin olive oil

4 big ripe tomatoes, roasted and pealed

1 small red bell pepper, roasted and peeled

1 medium white onion, minced

4 whole garlic cloves, bruised with the skin

5 cups chicken stock

4 tablespoons cilantro leaves

1/2 teaspoon cumin

Salt and pepper to taste

For garnish:

1 avocado, ripe but firm, pealed and cubed

1/2 teaspoon cilantro

3 tablespoons yogurt cheese

Directions

Preheat oven at 350 F. Brush a little olive oil on a baking sheet. Roast the tomatoes, garlic and red pepper for 20 minutes. Heat a pot over medium low heat and cook the onion until soft, about 8 minutes. Take out the tray form the oven and allow the ingredients to cool off before peeling. Transfer the tomatoes, pepper, garlic and juices released during roasting to a blender and mix together with the cooked onion, cilantro and 1 cup chicken stock. Return the contents back into the stockpot, add the rest of the stock and season with salt and pepper. Simmer uncovered until ready to eat. Serve in soup bowls with avocado, yogurt cheese and a touch of fresh cilantro.

Note: This is a Mexican classic, and one of my favorite soups ever! I have made a few changes to make it suitable for the Yogurt Diet. You will therefore find that this tortilla soup has no tortillas. Shame on me!

Cream of Vegetable Soup

Ingredients

Extra virgin olive oil
1 carrot, cubed
1/2 onion, minced
2 leeks, white part only, thinly sliced
1 stalk celery, thinly sliced
1/4 cup red lentils, as a thickener
2 leek tops, to fill in with herbs
2 bay leaves
4 sprigs of thyme
 6 sprigs parsley
6 cups water, filtered
1 cup yogurt, Greek style
1 tablespoon parsley, chopped
1 teaspoon chives, chopped
Salt and pepper to taste

Directions

Bring a medium saucepan to medium low heat, cover the bottom with olive oil and cook the vegetables and lentils, stirring constantly, until the vegetables are soft, about 15 minutes. Insert the bay leaf, thyme and parsley inside each of the leek tops. Pour water into the saucepan; add the leek tops with the herbs and salt to taste. Bring to a boil, then reduce the heat immediately and simmer covered for 20 minutes.
Discard the herbs. Transfer the soup to a blender and puree in small batches. Return to the saucepan and keep at a simmer until ready to use, about 10 minutes. Serve in soup plates with a dollop of yogurt and sprinkle with chives.

Cream of Asparagus

Ingredients

20 thick green asparagus, trimmed and bottoms peeled
Extra virgin olive oil
3 cups chicken stock
1 cup water, filtered
1 white onion, peeled and halved
1 leek, separate white and green parts
2 thyme sprigs
1 bay leaf
4 chives, thinly chopped for garnish
4 tablespoons heavy cream yogurt
Salt and pepper to taste

Directions

Peel the tough skin on the bottom of the asparagus. Cut the tips and set aside. In a medium saucepan, bring the chicken stock and water with a pinch of salt to a boil and submerge the asparagus tips for 5 minutes. Take them out with a slotted spoon and set aside. In the same saucepan, cook the onion, both parts of the leek, thyme sprigs, bay leave and 3 tablespoons olive oil for 15 minutes. Add the asparagus o the saucepan and cook for another 15 minutes. Discard the green leaves of the leek, thyme and bay leaf. Mix the vegetables in batches in an electric blender with 1 cup of the stock. Return to the saucepan along with the asparagus tips, season to taste and simmer. Serve with a dollop of yogurt and minced chives. You may eat chilled or warm.

Minty Green Pea Soup

Ingredients

2 cups fresh, shelled English peas or frozen petite peas
Extra virgin olive oil
1 small head Boston lettuce, sliced
6 spring onions, white and light green parts only, sliced
1/4 cup mint leaves
1 bay leaf
4 cups water, filtered
1 splash lime juice
Salt and pepper to taste
1/2 cup drained yogurt
1tablespoon fresh dill
Salt and pepper to taste

Directions

Cover the bottom of a large saucepan over medium heat with olive oil, and sauté the green onions until soft, about 8 minutes. Add the lettuce and cook for another 5 minutes. Pour the water and add the peas with the bay leaf. Reduce heat to low, simmer covered for 20 minutes. Remove from the heat and let it cool off.

Transfer the contents to a blender; add the mint leaves and lime juice, and purée, working in batches, until smooth and creamy. Season to taste. Refrigerate and serve chilled on soup plates with a dollop of yogurt and sprinkle with dill and a few drops of olive oil.

Watercress Summer Soup

Ingredients

2 robust bunches water cress leaves
Extra virgin olive oil
1/2 celery root, peeled and thinly sliced
1 yellow onion, peeled and minced
1 clove garlic
4 cups water, filtered
2 Persian cucumbers, thinly sliced
1/2 teaspoon cumin
Salt and pepper to taste

Directions

Separate the watercress leaves from its stems. Heat a large saucepan over medium low heat, cover with olive oil and sauté onions and celery root until barely soft, about 10 minutes. Pour water, add cumin, salt and pepper and simmer uncovered for 10 minutes. Remove the soup from the heat and submerge the watercress. Cover and let it steep for 5 minutes. Blend in an electric mixer in very small batches. Cool in the refrigerator and serve with cucumber slices.

Mom's Cucumber Yogurt Soup

Ingredients

5 Persian cucumbers or 1 large English cucumber

2.5 cups whole natural yogurt

2 parsley sprigs

8 mint leaves

2 small garlic cloves

1/2 celery, peeled

1 1/2 cups filtered water

2 tablespoons raw pine nuts

1/2 tablespoon dill

Salt and pepper, to taste

Directions

In a blender mix the first 7 ingredients together. Use water as needed to achieve a creamy and silky consistency. Serve chilled, sprinkled with pine nuts, or other raw nuts, and dill.

Thai Chicken Soup

Ingredients

1 chicken carcass with 2 whole legs, from leftovers

1 1/3 quarts water, filtered

1 medium onion, peeled and whole

1 stalk lemon grass, white part only, halved lengthwise

3 kaffir lime leaves, fresh or dried

1 (3-inch) piece fresh ginger, peeled

5 garlic cloves, crushed with the skin on

1 lime, quartered

1/4 cup chopped fresh cilantro leaves

Salt and pepper to taste

Directions

Use the leftover carcass and legs from the previous day's roasted chicken. Discard the contents from inside the chicken's cavity; place the carcass with the legs in a large stockpot and cover generously with water. Add the onion, lemon grass, kaffir lime leaves, ginger, garlic and salt. Bring to a rapid boil, immediately lower heat to a slow simmer and cook uncovered for 2 hours.

Carefully strain the stock through a fine sieve into another pot to separate the liquid from the solids. Hand-shred the leg meat and add it to the stock. Stir in the coconut oil and simmer for 5 minutes.

Serve hot, sprinkled with cilantro, fresh cracked pepper and a lime wedge on the side.

Note: The directions to make this easy soup recipe are to use the leftovers from the roasted chicken made the day before. Alternatively, you may also make this soup with 2 whole legs of chicken and 1 lb chicken wings.

GRAINS AND DRIED BEANS

How to Cook Dried Beans and Legumes

1. Remove any little stones, moldy and wrinkled beans.
2. Put the beans in a colander and rinse them well under cool running water
3. Transfer the beans or legumes to a large pot and cover with cold filtered water. Soak the beans over night, or at least four hours prior to cooking. This will have various effects. Among others, it will activate the enzymes present in the dried beans and it will also get rid of gas causing compounds. Discard any beans that come to the surface.
4. Throw away the soaking water and give the beans a quick rinse.
5. In a large stockpot, combine the legumes with the cooking liquid and any herbs you wish. The ratio of beans to liquid is generally 1 quart of liquid to 8 Oz of beans.
6. Bring to a full boil.
7. Reduce to medium low and cook uncovered until done. Add more liquid if necessary. If the legumes absorb all the liquid they will scorch.
8. Add salt near the end of cooking time.
9. Drain the beans or let them cool off in the cooking liquid.
10. Use them in salads or serve as soup.

Notes:

The amount of liquid and cooking time required for beans depends on the type and size. Between 25 and 45 minutes. Bite into a bean to check for doneness. Beans should be completely covered with liquid at all times. Add more liquid if necessary during cooking. Stir occasionally to prevent scorching. Lentils, split peas and black-eyed peas do not need to be presoaked.

Cooking Ratios and Times for Grains

1 cup of each dried grain yields approximately 4 servings when cooked

Type	Ratio of grain to liquid (cups)	Cooking Time
Millet	1:2	30-35 minutes
Oat, whole grain	1:2	45 minutes-1 hour
Oat, rolled	1:3	25 minutes
Rice, basmati and jasmine	1:11/2	25 minutes
Rice, Black or red	1:1/2	25 minutes
Rice, Long-grain, brown	1:2	30 minutes
Rice, short-grain, brown	1:2	30 minutes
Rice, wild	1:2	30-45 minutes
Quinoa	1:11/2	15-20 minutes
Amaranth	1:11/2	15-20 minutes

Coconut Rice

Ingredients

Serves 4

1 cup whole grain rice of choice

1/2 tablespoon extra virgin olive oil

1/2 tablespoon coconut oil

2 cups filtered water

Salt to taste

Directions

Heat the olive and coconut oils in a heavy bottomed pot over medium heat. Add the rice and sauté for 5 minutes, stirring constantly, until well coated. Add the water and season with salt. Bring to a boil and cover. Lower the heat and simmer until the grains are tender, about 25-30 minutes. Remove from the heat and let stand for 5 minutes. Uncover and fluff with a fork.

Brown Rice Pilaf with Pecans and Scallions

Ingredients

Serves 4

1 cup brown basmati rice

1 tablespoon extra virgin olive oil

1 shallot, minced

2 cups chicken stock or filtered water

Chopped toasted pecans

2 tablespoons green onions, white part only, thinly sliced

Salt and pepper to taste

Directions

Heat the olive oil in a heavy-bottomed pot over medium heat. Add the shallot and sweat, stirring frequently, until translucent, about 5 minutes. Add the rice and sauté for 5 minutes, stirring constantly, until well coated. Add the liquid, season with salt and stir once to prevent the rice from clumping together or sticking to the bottom. Bring to a boil and cover the pot. Lower the heat and simmer until the grains are tender, about 35 minutes. Remove from the heat and let stand for 5 minutes. Uncover and helping with a fork fold in the pecans and scallions, as the grains separate and release the steam. Salt and pepper to taste.

Cilantro-Lime Rice

Ingredients

Serves 4

1 cup brown long grain rice

1 tablespoon extra virgin olive oil

1 large shallot, minced

2 large garlic cloves, minced

2 cups chicken stock or filtered water

Juice of 1 lime

Grated zest of 1 lime

2 tablespoons minced cilantro

Salt and pepper to taste

Directions

Heat olive oil in a heavy-bottomed pot over medium heat. Add the shallot and sweat, stirring frequently, until translucent, about 2 minutes, then add the garlic and sauté for 45 seconds. Incorporate the rice and stir constantly, until well coated. Add the liquid to the rice and stir to prevent it from clumping together or sticking to the bottom. Bring to a boil and cover. Lower the heat and simmer until the grains are tender, about 30 minutes. Remove from the heat and let stand for 5 minutes. Uncover and using a fork, fluff to separate the grains and release the steam. Stir in the limejuice, lime zest and cilantro and season with salt and pepper to taste.

Basmati & Wild Rice Pilaf

Ingredients

Serves 4

1 cup basmati and wild rice mix

1 tablespoon extra virgin olive oil

4 tablespoons onion, diced

2 cups chicken stock or filtered water, heated

1 bay leaf

2 thyme sprigs

Salt and pepper to taste

Directions

Heat the olive oil in a heavy-bottomed pot over medium heat. Add the onions and sweat, stirring frequently, until translucent, about 5 minutes. Add the rice and sauté, stirring constantly, until well coated with oil. Add the liquid, bay leaf, thyme and season with salt. Stir to prevent the rice from clumping together. Bring to a boil, cover the pot, and simmer until the grains are tender, about 35 minutes. Remove from the heat and let stand for 5 minutes. Uncover and fluff with a fork to separate the grains and release the steam. Season to taste.

Quinoa Pilaf with Red and Yellow Peppers

Ingredients

Serves 4

1 cup quinoa

1 tablespoon extra virgin olive oil

1 large shallot, minced

1 large garlic clove, minced

2 cups chicken stock or filtered water

1 bay leaf

1 thyme sprig

1 diced roasted red pepper, diced

1 diced roasted yellow pepper, diced

Salt and pepper to taste

Directions

Roast peppers in the oven. Rinse the quinoa under cool running water to remove the grain's bitter coating. Let it drain. Heat the oil in a heavy-bottomed pot over medium heat. Add the shallots and garlic and sweat until translucent, about 2 minutes. Sauté the quinoa for 5 minutes, coat well, stirring constantly. Pour the liquid and add the bay leaf, thyme, and salt. Stir to prevent the quinoa from clumping or sticking to the bottom. Bring to a boil and cover the pot. Lower the heat and simmer until the grains are tender, about 20 minutes.

Remove form the heat and let stand for 5 minutes. Uncover and fluff using a fork to separate the grains and release the steam. Fold in the roasted peppers. Season to taste.

Couscous Salad

Ingredients

Ingredients

Serves 4

Serves 4

1 cup millet

6 tablespoons olive oil

2 tablespoon lemon juice

6 vine ripe tomatoes, seeded and diced

1/2 small Spanish onion, minced

1 Persian cucumber, diced

1/3 cup parsley, chopped

Salt and pepper to taste

Directions

Cook millet as directed (page 259). Fluff up with a fork, add olive oil, lemon, and mix well. Fold in the rest of the ingredients to make the salad. Season with salt and pepper to taste and serve at room temperature.

Saffron Rice

Ingredients

Serves 4

1 cup jasmine brown rice

Extra virgin olive oil

1 shallot, minced

1 1/2 cups water

1 big pinch saffron threads (about 20)

1 inch cinnamon stick

1 teaspoon cumin

Sea salt and pepper to taste

Directions

Heat the olive oil in a heavy-bottomed pot over medium heat. Add the shallot and sweat until translucent, stirring frequently, about 5 minutes. Add the rice and coat well with olive oil. Add water, saffron, cinnamon, cumin and salt. Stir to prevent the rice from clumping together. Bring to a boil and cover the pot. Lower the heat and simmer until the grains are tender, about 35 minutes. Remove from the heat and let stand for 5 minutes. Uncover, and fluff using a fork to separate the grains and release the steam. Season to taste.

Quinoa Tabbouleh

Ingredients

Serves 4

1cup quinoa or millet

2/3 cups extra virgin olive oil, more if needed

Juice of 1 lemon

1/4 cup parsley leaves, finely chopped

1/8 cup mint leaves, finely chopped

4 scallions, tops trimmed and sliced thinly

2 flavorful tomatoes, seeded and diced

Salt and pepper to taste

Directions

Cook the grain following directions (page 259). Put the quinoa or millet in a serving dish and pour over the lemon juice, olive oil, salt and pepper to taste. Toss with two forks to loosen up. Mix together with the parsley, mint, scallions and tomatoes. Serve at room temperature.

Stewed chickpeas with tomato and zucchini

Ingredients

Serves 4

2 cups chickpeas, cooked

1 cup cooking liquid, reserved form chickpeas

Extra virgin olive oil

2 garlic cloves, minced

1 large zucchini, diced

1 cup cherry tomatoes, halved

2 tablespoons cilantro, chopped

Fresh lime juice, to taste

Salt and pepper, to taste

Directions

Cook the chickpeas as directed (page 258) Reserve 1 cup of the cooking liquid. Drain the chickpeas in a colander and discard any lose skins. Cover the bottom of a pan with olive oil over medium heat and sauté garlic for 45 seconds. Add zucchini and cherry tomatoes and cook until zucchini is tender, about 10 minutes. Add the chickpeas and cooking liquid. Stew for 15 minutes. Make sure there's enough liquid to keep them moist. Add the cilantro and lime juice. Season to taste.

Braised Lentils with Eggplant

Ingredients

Serves 4

1 cup brown lentils

Extra virgin olive oil

4 cups chicken stock or filtered water, as needed

1 small onion, minced

2 garlic cloves, minced

1/2 large eggplant, diced

1/2 teaspoon curry powder

Grated lemon zest of 1 lemon

Salt and pepper to taste.

Directions

Cook lentils as directed (page 258). Preheat the oven at 350°F. Heat the oil in a Dutch oven or heavy bottom pot over medium heat, cover the bottom with olive oil and sauté the onions until tender and lightly golden, about 8 minutes. Add the garlic and cook for 45 seconds, stirring frequently. Stir in the eggplant and coat evenly with oil. Add the cinnamon, turmeric and lemon zest. Cook for 8 minutes. Add the cooked lentils and enough cooking liquid to moisten them well. Cover and place in the oven. Braise for 15 minutes, until the eggplant is completely tender. Season to taste.

Humus

Ingredients

Serves 4

1cup chickpeas

2 tablespoons olive oil, plus more to drizzle on top

1 bay leaf

4 garlic cloves, 2 unpeeled and crushed, 2 pealed

1/2 cup cooking liquid, from chickpeas

4 tablespoons sesame seeds

1 tablespoon lemon juice, plus more if needed

Zest of 1/2 orange

1 pinch cumin

3 tablespoons yogurt

Salt and pepper to taste

5 large carrots, cut in 2-inch sticks

5 celery stalks, cut in 2-inch sticks

Directions

Cook the chickpeas (page 258) and add 1 bay leaf, and 2 crushed garlic cloves to the cooking liquid. Drain the chickpeas, and save 1/2 cup of the cooking liquid.

In the food processor add the chickpeas, garlic, 3 tablespoons cooking liquid, olive oil, lemon juice, orange zest, sesame seeds, a pinch of cumin and salt. Blend well until creamy. Add more liquid if you too thick, then add yogurt and pepper. Blend one more time. Refrigerate. Take out 1 hour before serving and drizzle generously with olive oil. Serve with carrot and celery sticks.

Breakfast Oatmeal

Ingredients

Serves 2

1/2 cup rolled oats

1 1/2 cups filtered water

1 large pinch salt

Agave, to taste

2 teaspoons butter, or coconut butter

Cinnamon (optional)

Directions

In a saucepan, bring the oats with salt to a boil. Quickly reduce heat and simmer uncovered, stirring occasionally for 25 minutes until creamy. Serve on individual bowls and add butter and agave. Blend the flavors together and sprinkle with cinnamon or crushed nuts if desired.

Breakfast Black Rice

Ingredients

Serves 2

1/2 cup black rice

2 cups water, filtered

Pinch of salt

Agave, to taste

2 heaping teaspoons coconut butter

Directions

Bring the rice to a boil, add a pinch of salt, cover and lower to a simmer. Cook for 25 minutes. Serve on individual bowls with agave nectar and coconut butter. Stir well.

SAUCES

Salsa

Serves 4

3 vine ripe tomatoes, seeded and diced

1/3 cup white onions, minced

1 tablespoon cilantro, chopped

1 jalapeño pepper, seeded and minced

2 tablespoons lime juice

3 tablespoons extra virgin olive oil

Salt and pepper to taste

Directions

Combine all the ingredients. Toss gently to mix the flavors together. Adjust the seasoning with salt and pepper to taste. Keep refrigerated until ready to use.

Guacamole

Ingredients

Makes 2 cups
2 avocados, ripe but firm
Juice of 2 limes
3 tablespoons jalapeño peppers, minced
3 green onions, white part only, sliced
2 tablespoons cilantro
Salt and pepper to taste

Directions

Cut the avocados in half, remove the pits and reserve for later. Scoop out the meet into a bowl and mash with a fork. Fold in the rest of the ingredients. Taste for seasoning and adjust with lime juice, salt and pepper. Add the pits to the guacamole until you're ready to serve. This is a little trick I learned from a good Mexican friend, who taught me that the pits prevent the guacamole from turning brown. Cover and refrigerate until ready to use.

Yogurt Sauce

Ingredients

Serves 2

1/2 cup rolled oats

1 1/2 cups filtered water

1 large pinch salt

Agave, to taste

2 teaspoons butter, or coconut butter

Cinnamon (optional)

Directions

Mix all ingredients in a bowl. Season to taste with salt and pepper. Dab a little paprika on top and drizzle a few drops of olive oil. Serve cold.

Serve as a side dish with chicken or lamb.

Mango Chutney

Serves 4

1 chopped mango

1 tablespoon jalapeño pepper, minced

1 small garlic clove, minced

1 teaspoon ginger, grated

1 teaspoon agave nectar

1 teaspoon limejuice

1/2 teaspoon turmeric

Salt and pepper, to taste

Directions

Combine all the ingredients together. Refrigerate until ready to use.

Mayonnaise

Serves 4

2 egg yolks

1/2 tablespoon dried mustard

3/4 cup extra virgin olive oil

Salt and pepper to taste

3/4 tablespoon lemon juice

Directions

Combine the yolk, water, lemon juice, and mustard in a bowl. Mix well with an electric mixer until the mixture is slightly foamy. Gradually add the olive oil constantly beating with the electric mixer, first a few drops at a time, growing into a thin stream, until the oil is incorporated and the mayonnaise is thick. Adjust the flavor with salt and lemon juice. Refrigerate the mayonnaise right away.

Chimichurri Sauce

Ingredients

Makes about 1 cup.

1 cup fresh Italian parsley leaves, minced

1/2 cup olive oil

1/3 cup lemon juice

1/2 lemon rind, grated

1/4 cup fresh cilantro leaves, minced

2 garlic cloves, peeled

3/4 teaspoon dried red pepper flakes

1/2 teaspoon ground cumin

1/2 teaspoon salt

Directions

Put all ingredients in a bowl and whisk until well mixed. Serve at room temperature. This sauce goes well with meat, lamb and chicken.

YOGURT RECIPES

Homemade Natural Yogurt

Ingredients

Makes 1-quart yogurt
1-quart (1 liter) whole milk (non-homogenized preferred)
3 tablespoons live active culture yogurt or one 5 ounce starter package
freeze dried bacteria

Directions

Improvise a double boiler. Fill up a saucepan or stockpot with water and fit a flameproof glass or stainless steel bowl on top touching the water. Fill up the bowl with whole milk and bring just to a boil. Stir frequently to prevent a layer from forming on the top.

Set aside and let cool off to about 110°F, stirring occasionally to prevent a film from forming. At this time mix in the starter together with one cup of the lukewarm milk and 3 tablespoons natural live active yogurt and pour back into the rest of the milk. If you're using a freeze-dried culture, follow directions on the package.

Preheat oven at 350°F for just 5 minutes. Turn the oven off, insert the bowl of milk and turn the oven light on. This will be your improvised incubator. Leave undisturbed between 6-8 hours. Do not move or insert anything inside, or the delicate fermentation process will get interrupted. Refrigerate for 5 hours before serving. If you opt for a yogurt maker instead, use as directed.

Greek Style Yogurt / Drained Yogurt

Ingredients

1 quart natural yogurt

Directions

Make yogurt as directed, using the recipe on top. Greek yogurt is simply drained yogurt, which consists on separating the solid milk contents from the liquids, known as whey.

Arrange a large mesh sieve (strainer) over a large bowl and cover with a cheesecloth. Pour in the yogurt and tie the 4 ends together as if making a little package. Strain the yogurt in the refrigerator for one day. Save the whey, an important milk protein packed with nutrients that has endless health benefits, and use it in smoothies, soups, and as a natural cure for many ailments. It keeps well in the refrigerator for up to one month.

Yogurt Cheese

Ingredients

1 quart natural yogurt

Directions

Follow the directions for Greek yogurt. Strain for 2 days with some type of heavy weight on top to drain all the liquid well. After 2 days, unwrap and mix with any herbs and spices of your choice. The possibilities are truly endless. Following is one recipe I make quite often to use in salads and as a snack.

Herbed Yogurt Cheese

Ingredients

1 cup yogurt cheese
1 garlic
2 sprigs fresh thyme
2 sprigs fresh rosemary
1/2 tablespoon chives
1/2 teaspoon sea salt
1/2 teaspoon black pepper, fresh milled

Directions

Mix all the ingredients together in a food processor or blender until it becomes creamy in consistency. Do not over blend. I like to make little balls and keep them in a tight sealed glass container drizzled with olive oil. Always ready to eat at a moments notice, as a snack or you can add it to your favorite salad.

SMOOTHIES AND DESSERTS

For the following recipes, always use plain natural yogurt of your choice, it can be Greek style or regular yogurt. If you desire, you may also substitute regular yogurt for natural kefir or even blend any of these choices of fermented milk products together. The rule is to always start with the purest yogurt possible, as you will be adding your own choice of fresh ingredients. The only equipment you will need to make the smoothies is a blender.

Pick and choose from the delicious recipes that follow and eat with each meal, they make wonderful deserts, snacks, and on the go pick me uppers.

Three yogurts a day keep the weight and doctor away!

Yogurt and fruit

Ingredients

Serves 1

5 oz natural yogurt

1/4 cup fresh fruit, cut into bite size pieces

Agave nectar to taste

2 tablespoons choice of nuts, optional

Directions

Place yogurt in a bowl, add the fruit and nuts and drizzle with agave

Lassi

Serves 4

1 1/2 cups natural yogurt

1/3 teaspoon ground cardamom

1/2 teaspoon cumin seeds

1/3 teaspoon sea salt

1 cup chilled filtered water

Directions

Mix all the ingredients together in a blender. Serve chilled.

Basic Fruit Smoothie

Ingredients

Serves 2
10-ounces natural yogurt
Juice of 2 Valencia oranges, fresh squeezed
1 teaspoon agave
1 cup fruit of your choice from the fruit list

Directions

Mix all the ingredients in an electric blender. Add 1 cup of ice if desired.

Note: With the ingredients above as a starting base, make your own creations using any seasonal fruits from the fruit list allowed to eat during the Yogurt Diet: peaches, nectarines, apples, apricots, cherries, tangerines, lemons, pomegranates, kumquats, persimmons, pears, mangoes, bananas, passion fruit, papaya, cherimoya, guava. And herbs: ginger, mint, cilantro, cumin, cocoa, matcha green tea...

Mango Orange Yogurt Smoothie

Ingredients

Serves 2

10-ounces natural yogurt

1 mango, pealed and pitted

Juice of 2 Valencia oranges, fresh squeezed

Juice of 1-inch piece ginger root

1 teaspoon agave

Directions

Mix all the ingredients together in a blender. Add 1 cup of ice if desired

Totally Orange Smoothie

Ingredients

Serves 2

10-ounce natural plain yogurt

Juice of 2 Valencia oranges, fresh squeezed

Zest of 1/2 orange

1 large carrot, peeled

1 pinch cumin

1/2 teaspoon orange flower water

Directions

Mix all the ingredients together in a blender. Reserve 1/2 teaspoon of the orange zest for garnish. Add ice if desired or place in the freezer for 15 minutes.

Rosewater almond yogurt

Ingredients

10-ounce yogurt
1/2 cup chilled filtered water
1/8 cup blanched raw almonds
1 teaspoon rosewater
1/3 teaspoon ground cardamom
1/2 teaspoon agave

Directions

Put all the ingredients in the blender and mix well. Serve chilled.

Following are variations of smoothies using cucumber as the focal ingredient. Cucumber possess a cleansing nature, therefore, the rest of the ingredients have been chosen to enhance the detoxifying effects of the smoothies. These ingredients are also very refreshing and soothing. You may drink these smoothies before or in between meals as a digestive tonic.

Cucumber Watercress Smoothie

Serves 2

10-ounce plain natural yogurt

1 Persian cucumber

1 handful of watercress leaves, about 20

1 teaspoon rose water

5 mint leaves

Dash lemon juice

Pinch sea salt

1/2 cup chilled filtered water

Directions

Put ingredients in a blender and mix well

Cucumber apple and celery smoothie

Ingredients

Serves 2

10-ounces natural yogurt

1/2 English cucumber, peeled and deseeded

1 green apple, peeled and cored

1/2 celery stalk, peeled

Squeeze of lime

6 mint leaves

Pinch salt

3/4 cup chilled filtered water

Directions

Put ingredients in a blender and mix well.

Cucumber Kiwi Lime Smoothie

Ingredients

10-ounces natural yogurt

2 small Persian cucumbers, peeled

1 kiwi, peeled

Lime juice of 1/2 lime

1/2 teaspoon ginger root juice

1/2 teaspoon agave

Directions

Put ingredients in a blender and mix well. Add 1 cup of ice if desired.

Cocoa coconut crunch

Ingredients

Serves 1

5-ounces natural yogurt

1/2 tablespoon raw cocoa

1/2 tablespoon coconut butter

1/3 tablespoon agave

3 drops vanilla extract

2 tablespoons hazelnuts, crushed

Directions

Mix ingredients together in a bowl with a spoon until well blended and creamy.
Fold in the hazelnuts at the end. Cool in the freezer for 30 minutes.

Chocomint Frozen Yogurt

Ingredients

Serves 1

5-ounces natural yogurt

1/2 tablespoons raw cocoa

8 mint leaves, minced

1/3 tablespoon agave, add more to taste

Directions

Mix ingredients together in a bowl with a spoon. Cool in the freezer for 30 minutes.

Cocoa Orange Blossom

Ingredients

Serves 2

10-ounces natural yogurt

1 tablespoon raw cocoa

1/2 orange with skin on, washed well and deseeded

Large pinch ground cinnamon

1 tablespoon agave

1 pinch salt

Directions

Mix ingredients together in a blender. Pour the contents into individual containers and cool in the freezer for 30 minutes.

Cocoa Mono Loco Smoothie

Serves 2

10-ounces natural yogurt

1 1/2 tablespoons raw cocoa

1 banana

1 tablespoon coconut butter

1 tablespoon agave

1 pinch nutmeg

Directions

Mix ingredients together in a blender. Add 1 cup of ice if desired or cool in the freezer for 20 minutes. Serve chilled in a glass.

Green Tea Frozen Yogurt

Ingredients

Serves 1

5-ounces natural yogurt

1 teaspoon matcha green tea powder

1/2 tablespoon agave

1 dash lime juice

Directions

Mix ingredients together in bowl with a spoon. Cool in the freezer for 30 minutes or simply eat right away.

Green Tea Mint Lemonade

Ingredients

Serves 1

5-ounces natural yogurt

1 teaspoon matcha green tea powder

5 fresh mint leaves

1 tablespoon lemon juice

1/8 cup filtered water, chilled

1/3 tablespoon agave, add more to taste

Directions

Mix ingredients together in a blender. Serve chilled

Green Tea Lemony Apple Frozen Yogurt

Ingredients

Serves 2

10-ounce natural yogurt

2 teaspoons matcha green tea powder

1 green apple, peeled and cored

Lemon zest of 1/2 lemon, well washed

1 tablespoon agave, add more to taste

Directions

Mix ingredients together in blender. Pour the contents into individual containers and cool in the freezer for 30 minutes.

REFERENCES

Allergy development and the intestinal microflora during the first year of life. Bengt Björkstén, Epp Sepp, Kaja Julge, Tiia Voor, Marika Mikelsaar. Journal of Allergy and Clinical Immunology (2001), Volume 108, Issue 4, Pages 516 – 520.

Bovee-Oudenhoven I; Termont D; Dekker R; Van der Meer R. **Calcium in milk and fermentation by yogurt bacteria increase the resistance of rats to Salmonella infection.** Gut (1996), 38(1), 59-65.

Brady LJ, Gallaher DD, Busta FF. **The role of probiotic cultures in the prevention of colon cancer.** Journal of Nutrition. (2000) 130:410S-414S.

Buchowski, Maciej S.; Simmons, Lorenza A.; Chen, Kong Y.; Flakoll, Paul J.; Mellen, Beverly G.; Turner, Ernest A. **Plasma leptin association with body composition and energy expenditure in sickle cell disease.** Journal of the American College of Nutrition (2000), 19(2), 228-236.

Cullen KW, Baranowski T, Baranowski L, Olvera N. **Social-environmental influences on children's diets:** results from focus groups with African-, Euro- and Mexican-American children and their parents. Health Educ Res 2000.

Cummings, John H.; Rombeau, John L.; Sakata, Takashi; Editors. **Physiological and Clinical Aspects of Short - Chain Fatty Acids.** (1995), 575 pp. Cambridge University Press.

Dannon Nutritopics: **Do fermented dairy products offer any protection against colorectal cancer?** No 26, March, 2004.

Dannon Nutritopics: **The health benefits of probiotics.** No 29, July, 2002.

Dannon Nutritopics: The three lines of defense in human intestine. 10th International congress of Bacteriology and Applied Microbilogy; Special topics. July 27th 2002. No 25, 2002.

Despres, Jean-Pierre; Lemieux, Isabelle. **Abdominal obesity and metabolic syndrome.** Nature (London, United Kingdom) (2006), 444(7121), 881-887.

Diet, nutrition, and the prevention of chronic disease. Report of a WHO study group. WHO Technical Report Series 797, Geneva 1990.

Dogs Lived 1.8 Years Longer On Low Calorie Diet: Gut Flora May Explain It. Imperial College London ScienceDaily Retrieved August 7, 2008, from http://www.sciencedaily.com⁻ /releases/2007/04/070419160140.htm.

Dunne, Colum; O'Mahony, Liam; Murphy, Lisa; Thornton, Gerardine; Morrissey, Darrin; O'Halloran, Sile; Feeney, Maria; Flynn, Sarah; Fitzgerald, Gerald; Daly, Charles; Kiely, Barry; O'Sullivan, Gerald C.; Shanahan, Fergus; Collins, J. Kevin. **In vitro selection criteria for probiotic bacteria of human origin: correlation with in vivo findings.** American Journal of Clinical Nutrition (2001), 73(2, Suppl.), 386S-392S.

Friedman, Jeffrey M.; Halaas, Jeffrey L. Leptin and the regulation of body weight in mammals. Nature (London) (1998), 395(6704), 763-770.

Gibson RG. **Fibre and effects on prbiotics (The prebiotic concept).** Clinical nutrition Supplements. (2004) 1(2) Pages 25-31.

Guarente, Leonard. **Sirtuins as potential targets for metabolic syndrome.** Nature (London, United Kingdom) (2006), 444(7121), 868-874.

Guarner F and Malagelada JR. **Gut flora in health and disease.** The Lancet. (2003) 361 (9356) 512-519.

Hamilton-Miller, J. M. T. **The role of probiotics in the treatment and prevention of Helicobacter pylori infection.** International Journal of Antimicrobial Agents (2003), 22(4), 360-366.

Hatakka K; Savilahti E; Ponka A; Meurman J H; Poussa T; Nase L; Saxelin M; Korpela R. **Effect of long term consumption of probiotic milk on infections in children attending day care centres : double blind , randomised trial.** BMJ (Clinical research ed.) (2001), 322(7298), 1327.

Hotamisligil, Goekhan S. **Inflammation and metabolic disorders.** Nature (London, United Kingdom) (2006), 444(7121), 860-867.

Kahn, Steven E.; Hull, Rebecca L.; Utzschneider, Kristina M. **Mechanisms linking obesity to insulin resistance and type 2 diabetes.** Nature (London, United Kingdom) (2006), 444(7121), 840-846.

Kalliomäki M, Isolauri E. **Role of intestinal flora in the development of allergy.** Curr Opin Allergy Clin Immunol 3(1):15-20, 2003.

Kepler C R; Hirons K P; McNeill J J; Tove S B **Intermediates and products of the biohydrogenation of linoleic acid by Butyrinvibrio fibrisolvens.** The Journal of biological chemistry (1966), 241(6), 1350-4.

Knight J. **Good bacteria in health and disease.** The Lancet (2004), Volume 361, Issue 9371, page 1831.

L. Näsea, K. Hatakkab, E. Savilahtic, M. Saxelinb, A. Pönkäe, T. Poussaf, R. Korpelab, J.H. Meurmana. **Effect of Long-Term Consumption of a Probiotic Bacterium, Lactobacillus rhamnosus GG, in Milk on Dental Caries and Caries Risk in Children.** Caries Res (2001) 35 (6) 412-420.

Ley, Ruth E.; Baeckhed, Fredrik; Turnbaugh, Peter; Lozupone, Catherine A.; Knight, Robin D.; Gordon, Jeffrey I. **Obesity alters gut microbial ecology.** Proceedings of the National Academy of Sciences of the United States of America (2005), 102(31), 11070-11075.

Life Extension Magazine, October 2000.

Lippincott Williams and Wilkins Bengt Björkstén. **Effects of intestinal microflora and the environment on the development of asthma and allergy.** (2004) 25(3-4) 257-270.

Marrugat, Jaume; Covas, Maria-Isabel; Fito, Montserrat; Schroeder, Helmut; Miro-Casas, Elisabet; Gimeno, Eva; Lopez-Sabater, M. Carmen; De La Torre, Rafael; Farre, Magi. **Effects of differing phenolic content in dietary olive oils on lipids and LDL oxidation : A randomized controlled trial.** European Journal of Nutrition (2004), 43(3), 140-147.

Martinez-Gonzalez Miguel Angel; Sanchez-Villegas Almudena **The emerging role of Mediterranean diets in cardiovascular epidemiology : monounsaturated fats, olive oil, red wine or the whole pattern?.** European journal of epidemiology (2004), 19(1), 9-13.

Marx, Jean. **Puzzling out the pains in the gut.** Science (Washington, DC, United States) (2007), 315(5808), 33-35.

Morton, G. J.; Cummings, D. E.; Baskin, D. G.; Barsh, G. S.; Schwartz, M. W. **Central nervous system control of food intake and body weight.** Nature (London, United Kingdom) (2006), 443(7109), 289-295.

Murphy, Kevin G.; Bloom, Stephen R. **Gut hormones and the regulation of energy homeostasis.** Nature (London, United Kingdom) (2006), 444(7121), 854-859.

Murphy, Kevin G.; Bloom, Stephen R. **Gut hormones and the regulation of energy homeostasis.** Nature (London, United Kingdom) (2006), 444(7121), 854-859.

Obesity: preventing and managing the global epidemic Report of a WHO Consultation Geneva, World Health Organization 2004.

Peter Parodi. **Anticarcinogenic nature of CLA in milk fat.** (Austral. J. Dairy Tech. (1994) 49, 93-97.

Pirkka V. Kirjavainen, Glenn R. Gibson. Healthy gut microflora and allergy: factors influencing development of the microbiota. Journal Annals of Medicine (1999) 31, (4) 288–292

Probiotics and The Hygiene Hypothesis: Harvard medical School, Division of Nutrition, A Case for Protective Nutrients April 3, 2006. Webcast available. *http://nutrition.med.harvard.edu/education/edu_exp_bio_conf.html.*

Riordan S M; McIver C J; Wakefield D; Duncombe V M; Thomas M C; Bolin T D **Small intestinal mucosal immunity and morphometry in luminal overgrowth of indigenous gut flora.** The American journal of gastroenterology (2001), 96(2), 494-500.

Sanders ME. **Considerations for use of probiotic bacteria to modulate human health.** Journal of Nutrition. (2000) 130:384s-390s.

Santora, Jamie E.; Palmquist, Donald L.; Roehrig, Karla L. **Trans - vaccenic acid is desaturated to conjugated linoleic acid in mice.** Journal of Nutrition (2000), 130(2), 208-215.

Sasaki, Makoto; Sakou, Toshinori; Joh, Takashi. **Effect on gut flora and blood**

glucose of synthesizing oligosaccharide enzymes. Shoka to Kyushu (2006), Volume Date 2005, 28(1), 79-81.

Sehat, Najibullah; Kramer, John K. G.; Mossoba, Magdi M.; Yurawecz, Martin P.; Roach, John A. G.; Eulitz, Klaus; Morehouse, Kim M.; Ku, Youh. **Identification of conjugated linoleic acid isomers in cheese by gas chromatography, silver ion high performance liquid chromatography and mass spectral reconstructed ion profiles. Comparison of chromatographic elution sequences.** Lipids (1998), 33(10), 963-971.

Seppo, Leena; Jauhiainen, Tiina; Poussa, Tuija; Korpela, Riitta. **A fermented milk high in bioactive peptides has a blood pressure - lowering effect in hypertensive subjects.** American Journal of Clinical Nutrition (2003), 77(2), 326-330.

Session: Short - chain fatty acids. Regulation of short – chain fatty acid production. Proceedings of the Nutrition Society (2003), 62(1), 67-72.

Sykora, Josef; Valeckova, Kristyna; Amlerova, Jana; Siala, Konrad; Dedek, Petr; Watkins, Stephen; Varvarovska, Jana; Stozicky, Frantisek; Pazdiora, Petr; Schwarz, Jan. **Effects of a Specially Designed Fermented Milk Product Containing Probiotic Lactobacillus casei DN -114 001 and the Eradication of H. pylori in Children: A Prospective Randomized Double-Blind Study.** Journal of Clinical Gastroenterology (2005), 39(8), 692-698.

Turnbaugh, Peter J.; Ley, Ruth E.; Mahowald, Michael A.; Magrini, Vincent; Mardis, Elaine R.; Gordon, Jeffrey I. **An obesity -associated gut microbiome with increased capacity for energy harvest.** Nature (London, United Kingdom) (2006), 444(7122), 1027-1031.

Van Gaal Luc F; Mertens Ilse L; De Block Christophe E **Mechanisms linking obesity with cardiovascular disease.** Nature (2006), 444(7121), 875-80.

Van Kessel Katherine; Assefi Nassim; Marrazzo Jeanne; Eckert Linda. **Common complementary and alternative therapies for yeast vaginitis and bacterial vaginosis : a systematic review.** Obstetrical & gynecological survey (2003), 58(5), 351-8.

Weinbrenner, Tanja; Fito, Montserrat; de la Torre, Rafael; Saez, Guillermo T.; Rijken, Philip; Tormos, Carmen; Coolen, Stefan; Albaladejo, Magi Farre; Abanades,

Sergio; Schroder, Helmut; Marrugat, Jaume; Covas, Maria-Isabel. **Olive oils high in phenolic compounds modulate oxidative /antioxidative status in men.** Journal of Nutrition (2004), 134(9), 2314-2321.

Willett WC. **Diet and coronary heart disease.** Monographs in Epidemology and Biostatistics. (1990) 15, 341-379

Wollowski I, Rechkemmer G, Pool-Zobel BL. **Protective role of probiotics and prebiotics in colon cancer.** Am J Clin Nutr. (2001) 73:451s.

Wynne AG, McCartney Al, Brostoff J, Hudspith BN, Glenn GR and Gibson G. **An in vitro assessment of the effects of broad-spectrum antibiotics on the human gut microflora and concomitant isolation of a Lactobacillus plantarum with anti-Candida activities.** Anaerobe. (2004) 10 (3) 165-169.

Xiong, Yumei; Miyamoto, Norimasa; Shibata, Kenji; Valasek, Mark A.; Motoike, Toshiyuki; Kedzierski, Rafal M.; Yanagisawa, Masashi. **Short - chain fatty acids stimulate leptin production in adipocytes through the G protein - coupled receptor GPR41.** Proceedings of the National Academy of Sciences of the United States of America (2004), 101(4), 1045-1050.

BOOKS

Balch, Phyllis A. (2000). *Prescription for Nutritional Healing.* Avery.

Brudnak, Mark A. (2003). *The Probiotic Solution.* Dragon Door Publications.

Burton Goldberg Group, (2002). *Alternative Medicine.* Celestial Arts.

Carroll, Ricki (2003). *Making Cheese, Butter and Yogurt.* A Storey Country Wisdom bulletin.

Chapell, James (2005). *A Promise Made, a Promise Kept.* BL publications.

Crook, William G. (1986). *The Yeast Connection: A Medical Breakthrough.* Professional Books.

David, Marc (1991). *Nourishing Wisdom.* Bell Tower.

Dowhower Karpa, Kelly (2003). *Bacteria for Breakfast.* Trafford publishing.

Enig, Mary G. (2000) *Know Your Fats: The Complete Primer for Understanding the Nutrition of Fats, Oils, and Cholesterol.* Bethesda Press. www.westonaprice.org

Fallon, Sally. **Nourishing Traditions.** New Trends Publishing.
http://www.westonaprice.org

Gittleman, Ann Louise (1999). *Eat Fat, Lose Weight.* Keats Publishing.

Hobbs, Christopher (1986, 2002). *Natural Therapy for Your Liver.* Avery.

Pitchford, Paul (2002). *Healing With Hole Foods.* North Atlantic Books.

Ravnskof, Uffe (2000). *The Cholesterol Myths.* New Trends Publishing.

Santillo, Humbart (1987). *Food Enzymes: Missing Link to Radiant Health.* Hohm Press.

Schmid, Ron (2003). *The Untold Story of Milk.* New Trends Publishing.

Sizer, Frances and Whitney, Ellie (2006). *Nutrition Concepts and Controversies.* Thomson Wadsworth.

Strand, Ray D. (2003). *Death by Prescription: The Shocking Truth Behind an Overmedicated Nation.* Thomas Nelson Pubublishers.

Taller, Herman (1961). *Calories Don't Count.* Simon and Schuster.

Trenev, Natasha (1998). *Probiotics: Nature's Internal Healers.* Health & Fitness Avery.

Truss, C. Orian (1982). *The Missing Diagnosis.* The Missing Diagnosis, Inc.

Zimmer, Carl (2001). *Parasite Rex: Inside the Bizarre World of Nature's Most Dangerous Creatures.* Simon and Schuster. *http://www.carlzimmer.com*

Ana Luque is a food coach and holistic chef who is rapidly becoming known internationally as "the yogurt expert." She is a pioneer in promoting yogurt as the star ingredient for an entire diet and lifestyle, one that stresses the great importance of a healthy and balanced gut flora to promote weight loss and health. Ana has traveled around the globe to study various traditional cuisines in her search for answers to resolving the obesity and health crises that afflict our society today. After many years of painstaking research she has concluded that the one important food missing in our modern diet is indeed probiotic yogurt. Ana's goal is to raise health awareness and stop the obesity epidemic that is overtaking our population by creating a yogurt culture in America. Ms Luque is also a public speaker and writer who is changing the lives of those touched by her passion, advice and natural recipes, all geared to promoting total health and well-being.

Ana shares her time between Los Angeles, and various cities in Europe. She is available to clients for private and group coaching in person and over the phone anywhere in the world.

To contact her go to her website www.analuque.com

Bill Gutman has been a freelance writer for some three decades. In that time, he has written numerous books, both non-fiction and fiction. Many have been in the sports field, but he has always put an emphasis on dealing with various personalities of interest, as well as on biography and sports history. He enjoys writing about sports, music, history, health and nutrition.

Some notable books include a biography of Magic Johnson (Magic, More Than A Legend); *The Giants Win the Pennant! The Giants Win the Pennant!*, an autobiography with Bobby Thomson and recreation of the 1951 pennant race between the New York Giants and Brooklyn Dodgers; *Parcells, A Biography*; and *Won For All*, the story of the New England Patriots 2001 Super Bowl season, written in collaboration with former All-Pro linebacker and current Patriots linebackers coach Pepper Johnson.

The author has also worked with football icon John Madden on *John Madden's Heroes of Football, The Story of America's Game*; and with former Red Sox and Rangers manager Kevin Kennedy on *Twice Around the Bases*. His lifelong interest in music and jazz was reflected in *Duke: The Musical Life of Duke Ellington*; and his most recent book is *What If the Babe Had Kept His Red Sox*, which talks about alternate histories from the world of sports.

Bill Gutman was born in New York City and currently lives in New York State.

Printed in the United States
140644LV00002B/1/P

9 780615 241050